The Natural Intelligence of Stem Cells

The Natural Intelligence of Stem Cells

The Story of a Breakthrough Discovery: Unlocking the Universal Language of Plant and Human Stem Cells to Regenerate and Rejuvenate

NATHAN NEWMAN, MD

The Journey of a Unicorn Doctor on a Global Mission to Cultivate Stem Cell Culture

The Natural Intelligence of Stem Cells: The Story of a Breakthrough Discovery: Unlocking the Universal Language of Plant and Human Stem Cells to Regenerate and Rejuvenate.

Innovated by Nathan Newman, MD

ISBN (print): 9798218637507
ISBN (ebook): 9798218637514

Production Services: Happenstance Type-O-Rama

Printed in the United States of America

With gratitude to God, and to:

My parents, Tajy and Dr. Samuel Newman, and my brother, Andre of blessed memory, who valued education and led by example of wisdom, courage, and compassion.

My dearest sister, Ziba Danielpour, and brother, Dr. Armand Newman, for their steadfast love and guidance throughout my life.

My beloved wife, Rinat, whose unwavering support, love, and dedication to our family have been my greatest anchor. You have stood by me through every challenge, embracing my dreams as your own and guiding them to life with your vision. For your wisdom, encouragement, and quiet strength as a partner, I am forever grateful.

My teachers and mentors, who instilled in me the courage to challenge conventions and seek out the resources necessary for discovery.

Maya Bodow, our brilliant CEO and COO, whose unwavering loyalty and exceptional leadership has been vital in building an extraordinary team and operation.

Dodanim Talavera, MD, PhD, our capable CSO, whose dedication and skills have helped to develop and patent our stem cell–derived platform technology.

My patients, whose trust in me is both humbling and inspiring, and who motivate me to continually find solutions and innovate.

Contents

Acknowledgments

To my extraordinary and dedicated medical and scientific team, who turn vision into reality:

Maya Bodow, MS, CEO

Jimmy Taus, Esq.

Nualla Rogowski, RN

Assaf Zemah, PhD

Meirav Bar-Yosef

Jenny Richey

Rinat Newman, CVO

Dodanim Talavera, MD, PhD, CSO

Marcelo Rotsztejn

Rosa Vargas, MA

Bong-Seop Lee, PhD

Ariyah Cohen

Your contributions are invaluable, and I am forever grateful for your commitment to our mission.

To Billie Fitzpatrick and Gail Sagel for your outstanding talent, wisdom, and dedication in editing this book and bringing it to life.

Introduction

As a doctor, I've always been fascinated by the body's ability to heal itself. But over the years, I've come to realize that this natural intelligence within us holds even greater potential than we ever imagined. My journey into the world of stem cells began with a simple yet profound question: What if we could harness the body's own regenerative power to heal and to rejuvenate?

This question led me to develop the Stem Cell Lift, a revolutionary procedure that utilizes the regenerative properties of your own stem cells to restore youthful vitality and enhance your overall well-being. In this book, I want to share with you the science and the technique behind the Stem Cell Lift, and the stories of the countless patients whose lives have been transformed by it. These are people who, like you, were searching for more than just a cosmetic fix; they were seeking a way to feel as vibrant on the outside as they did on the inside.

Seeking to help others and share the healing promise of stem cells beyond the scope of my clinic also inspired me to establish my research lab, where we've made groundbreaking discoveries. One of these advances is the development of *Consortia Factors(CFx)*, an extraordinary consortium of bioactive molecules that work together to balance, enhance, and guide your body's natural ability to heal, renew, and rejuvenate.

This patented technology to produce CFx represents a paradigm shift in healthcare. By integrating these factors into our STEM products we're not just enhancing cosmetic outcomes; we're pioneering a new approach to medicine that targets the root causes of aging and disease, offering unprecedented possibilities for regeneration and overall wellness. CFx has the potential to transform how we approach health, offering treatments that are more effective, personalized, and holistic.

In this book, I'm excited to share with you the science behind these innovations and how they can help you achieve the results you've been dreaming of. You'll learn how stem cells and CFx work together, why they're so powerful, and how this technology is poised to revolutionize the future of healthcare. Even more than that, I hope you'll come away with a deeper understanding of how these advancements can empower you to make educated decisions in regard to your own aging process, enhancing your appearance and, more importantly, your overall quality of life.

My philosophy of care is simple: every person is unique, and so is your journey to wellness. This personalized approach is at the heart of everything I do, and it's why the Stem Cell Lift and the STEM technology have become a cornerstone of my practice. It's about more than just turning back the clock—it's about helping you live your life to the fullest, with confidence, energy, and a real renewed sense of self.

Thank you for joining me on this journey. I'm excited to share with you the incredible potential of stem cells and how Stem Cell Therapy and STEM technology can help you live a life that's not just longer in quantity, but better in quality.

PART I

The Regenerative Power of Stem Cells

"Every person deserves not just to be treated, but to be truly cared for."

—DR. NATHAN NEWMAN

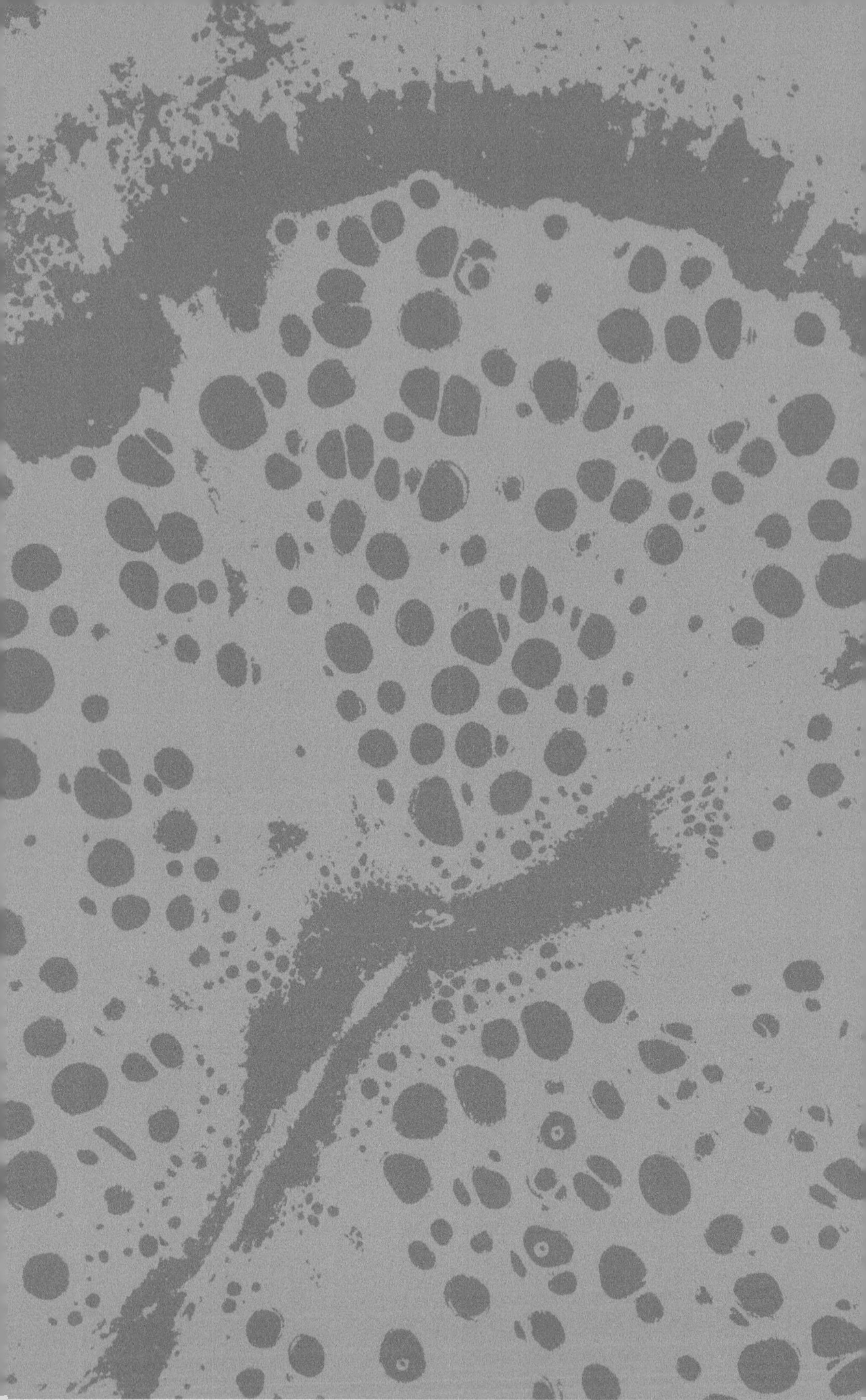

1
Harnessing the Healing Power of Creation

In order to appreciate the regenerative power of stem cells, it's helpful to understand what they are. Stem cells are called "mother cells" in Spanish, as they are an essential powerhouse of the body. As soon as a human embryo is formed, the body begins to grow in large part because of the action of embryonic stem cells (omnipotent cells). These powerful cells signal the growth and formation of the embryo. During the process of embryogenesis, cells develop into cell layers (including the endoderm, mesoderm, and ectoderm), which further develop into the various cells, organs, and tissues of the growing fetus, and later into the adult organism. As embryonic stem cells differentiate into specialized cell types, tissue or adult stem cells (also referred to as pluripotent stem cells) are produced within each organ and structure. These adult stem cells are tasked with the maintenance, repair, and renewal of all of our body structures.

Stem cells can be distinguished from other cells in the body in three important ways:

- They are undifferentiated (unspecialized), which means they have the ability to become different types of cells, depending on their environment. If a stem cell migrates or is injected into bone, the cells become bone; if they are transferred into the muscle, they become muscle cells; and so on. Scientists call this feature *pluripotency*.

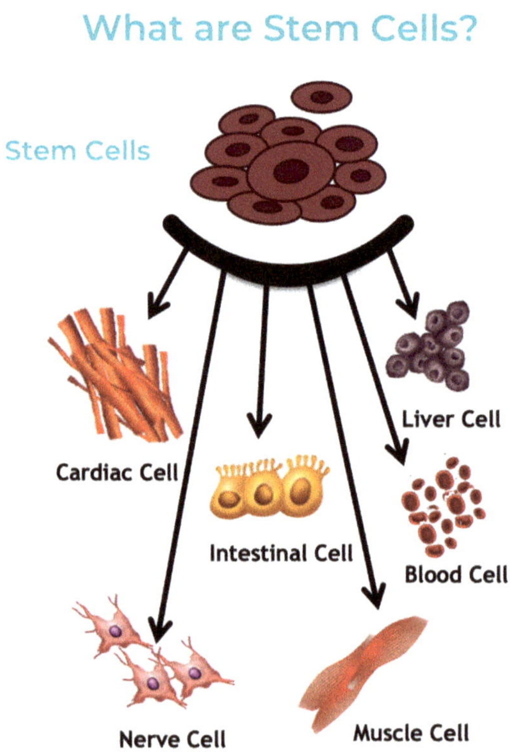

Stem cells' ability to transform into specific cell types

- They have the ability to self-renew and self-replicate while remaining undifferentiated. This means that they can divide and re-enter the cell cycle long-term, although this process is tightly regulated within the tissue.
- Most significantly, stem cells possess the innate ability to repair and regenerate tissue, which is why they are so powerful as healing agents.

In other words, stem cells are like soldiers: you put them in place, and they carry out the orders based upon their surroundings.

In addition, there are generally three different types of stem cells: embryonic stem cells, tissue (or adult) stem cells, and induced pluripotent stem cells (iPSCs), which act like embryonic stem cells. Tissue

The Unique Attributes of Stem Cells

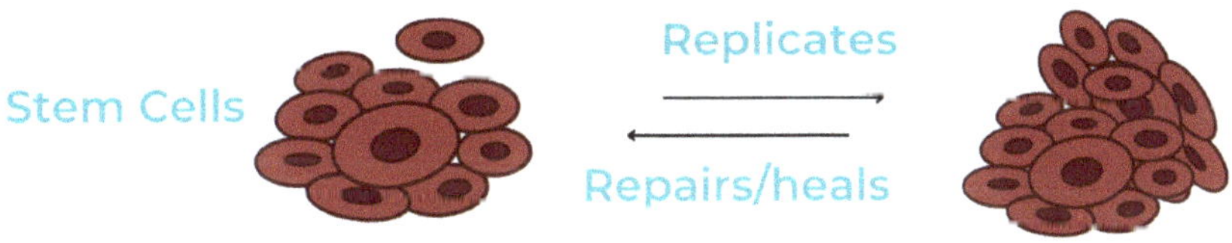

Self Renewal
Ability to make more stem cells

Pluripotent Differentiation
Ability to become different cell types

Repair & Regenerate
Ability to restore function to tissue

The unique properties that make stem cells so powerful

stem cells are characterized by being undifferentiated and able to self-renew. They are found throughout the tissues of the body, and though they are affected by aging, they are present throughout your lifetime. The function of adult stem cells is to enable the healing, growth, and replacement of cells that are lost or used up in the course of daily living, which explains why there are various types of stem cells, including:

- Mesenchymal stem cells, which differentiate into tissues such as bone, cartilage, and fat cells.
- Neural cells, which play an important role in neurogenesis (the process of forming new neurons).
- Hematopoietic stem cells, which help develop blood cells, including red and white blood cells and platelets.
- Skin stem cells, which are precursors to keratinocytes that form the protective layer of skin.

Initially, stem cell research focused on embryonic stem cells. However, embryonic stem cell therapy presented many challenges and was fraught with unwanted complications. One complication was the formation of teratomas (tumors composed of different body parts such as teeth, hair, and bone) in places where it was injected into the body. This reaction was the result of the omnipotent cells trying to create a human being. In addition, there were (and still are) ethical concerns over the use of embryonic stem cells, as they have the potential for life. These limitations in the use of embryonic stem cells for clinical use redirected researchers.

During the 1950s, researchers were conducting allogeneic bone marrow transplantation, a procedure that takes bone marrow blood from one patient and introduces it into another patient. These patients have to have a close human leukocyte antigen (HLA) match to prevent graft-versus-host disease (GVHD), where the newly introduced cells from a donor view the recipient cells as foreign and attack the recipient's tissues and organs, making the recipient ill. However, in the 1970s scientists discovered that the bone marrow contains a type of adult stem cell called mesenchymal stem cell. Later, they learned that these stem cells may have the ability to treat GVHD. From this technology came cord blood transplantation, in which cord blood is collected from the umbilical cord during childbirth. This procedure has been used in experimental treatments and for allogeneic hematopoietic stem cell transplantation (bone marrow transplantation).

While there were advances in embryonic research and hematopoietic stem cell transplantation, there was little knowledge about any other tissue stem cells until around the year 2000. In fact, the prevailing belief was that certain cells, such as fat and brain cells, were created during fetal development and did not change in number over our lifetime, so any damage to these cells would be permanent. This all changed as scientists discovered stem cells in just about every organ in the body. This discovery ushered in a new era in medicine and transformed our understanding of how the body works.

Today we know that tissue stem cells have the power not only to heal tissue after injury or disease, but also to renew every cell in the body, including bone, joints, skin, muscle, and brain cells. The medical

Allogeneic vs. Autologous Stem Cells

Allogeneic transplant Cells are taken from one individual and placed into other individuals.

Autologous transplant Cells are taken from an individual and placed back into that person.

field's knowledge of tissue stem cells has grown exponentially, in particular how they can be utilized to address musculoskeletal diseases, GI conditions, skin diseases, nervous disorders, and lung and heart disease. Research also showed how tissue stem cells' capacity to differentiate into multiple types of cells plays an important role in the regulation of the immune system, which points to enormous potential for preventing diseases altogether.

In 2006, scientists discovered that it's possible to create—or induce—pluripotent stem cells in vitro in the laboratory setting. Induced pluripotent stem cells (iPSCs) are cells that are genetically reprogrammed from somatic cells (cells derived from other types of cells of the body, such as skin or blood cells) back into an embryonic-like pluripotent state, making them a rich source of stem cells that may be used therapeutically. For example, iPSCs can be reprogrammed to become beta islet cells to treat diabetes, blood cells free of cancer cells to treat a leukemia patient, or neurons to treat neurological disorders. The discovery of iPSCs meant that scientists could now create (i.e., induce) adult stem cells in laboratory conditions and experiment to understand more about these fascinating feats of nature.

Although tissue stem cells can be found in every part of the body, they are most abundant in the adipose (fat) tissue, making those the easiest to access, collect, and use—without the need to multiply them in the lab—in the clinical setting.

It may be helpful to think about stem cells as an ever-giving source of renewal: they facilitate healing by bringing the body back into a more stable state when it becomes imbalanced due to any number of reasons—a trauma or injury, invasive medical treatments such as radiation or chemotherapy, a virus or bacterial infection, a cytokine storm as we saw with the COVID-19 epidemic, or any number of environmental insults or assaults, from air pollution to exposure to harsh chemicals. The central directive of our physiology is homeostasis: every cell and system in our body is programmed to return to a state of balance when it encounters a stressor, internal or external. Sometimes this drive toward homeostasis creates unwanted results and diminishes function in other areas of the body or speeds up aging and makes people more prone to disease. However, when autologous stem cells (the stem cells of a person's own body) are systematically reintroduced, they bring the body back into homeostatic balance. Further, stem cells work in lock-step with a patient's own immune system, giving it what it needs to heal holistically. The process of regaining and maintaining homeostasis is key to living a long, healthy life.

Discovering the Richest Source of Stem Cells: Fat

In my dermatology training, I had learned and specialized mostly in skin, hair, nails, and fat. Fat is one of the largest tissues in the human body, and it became a very important part of my dermatological studies and research, as I began learning to do common procedures in which fat was removed from one part of the body and placed in another part of the body for both reconstructive and cosmetic purposes. For instance, women who had gone through breast cancer treatment and had undergone a mastectomy were injected with fat tissue to reconstruct their breasts and correct contour deformities. This process is called *fat grafting* or *fat transfer*.

One of the first documented fat grafting procedures was performed in 1893 by Dr. Gustav Neuber, who took fat from his patient's arm and transferred it to the eye region to correct scarring from a bone infection. In 1895 Dr. Viktor Czerny transferred a lipoma to the breast to establish symmetry following a unilateral partial mastectomy. Following World War I, fat transfer procedures were used to help soldiers whose faces had been disfigured in combat. However, these early uses of fat were not always successful, as many times the fat cells used did not live long enough to graft into their new location and subsequently the cells were reabsorbed by the body.

During the next 100 years fat grafting was not very popular, as it had many complications and poor clinical results. Then, in 1985, Dr. Jeffrey A. Klein, a dermatologist, revolutionized liposuction surgery with his tumescent anesthesia technique, which used super-diluted local anesthesia to numb the area from where fat was to be taken with minimal damage to local tissues, such as nerves and blood vessels, resulting in only minimal surgical blood loss. Liposuction was thus transformed from being a very dangerous procedure to one of the safest and most popular procedures in the world. Since then, many advances have also been made in fat grafting techniques, making it a very safe and common procedure today.

During both my dermatology residency and cosmetic surgery fellowship, I was privileged to learn from many great surgeons who were utilizing different plastic surgery techniques for face and body enhancement. Many of these procedures, such as facial fat transfer, involved the use of fat as a medium for addressing cosmetic and dermatologic impairments.

Historically, surgeons used a method of fat removal that involved suctioning a patient's fat into a canister, pouring it into a sieve, and then washing the fat with saline (a sterile saltwater solution) to remove the blood and oil. The "cleaned" fat would then be scooped into a big syringe with a spoon and reinjected in large volume into the desired area of a patient's face, breast, buttock, or other area. This open-system procedure yielded poor results, with complications of lumpiness and hardness in the treated areas. During my training, physicians had begun using a newer technique that was considered less aggressive and involved removing the patient's fat directly through a syringe, which exerted less suction force on the fat cells, and then washing it with sterile solution in the confines of the syringe. This closed system minimized damage to the fat cells and thereby enabled better cells to be grafted. In addition, the fat was transferred from the big syringe to smaller syringes and injected in a layered and more precise fashion into the desired areas using a specially designed blunt cannula. The results were better but still unpredictable, with only 20 to 50 percent of the injected fat volume surviving and staying in place, most of it being reabsorbed by the body.

A Commitment to the Spirit of Inquiry: My Early Training

In Western medicine, we are taught to accept the status quo of science and continue to use best practices without really questioning the assumptions behind what we do and how we approach treatment. This attitude is embedded in how we are trained and what is expected of us as we work clinically and build our practices. My upbringing and personality have always led me to question standing assumptions and instead think critically, looking for better solutions and ways to solve problems or improve processes. Thus, I've always approached medicine as a physician and scientist and not as a technician. In that way, I've always considered myself a maverick. In addition, I always ensure that the benefits of any treatment must outweigh the risks for the safety and health of my patients. Following the mentorship of my father and our Jewish sages, I was looking for natural ways to work with the body, rather than manipulate it. My father taught me to "always listen to the patient; they know what they have." As a result, I respect and listen to my patients since most of the time they can describe best what they are suffering from and guide me to the source of their problem. I was also taught by my father and spiritual leaders to challenge the obvious, be curious, and cultivate original thinking. I naturally applied this life approach to my profession and have dedicated myself to always looking to learn more and seek out better, more effective approaches to healing. It is this spirit of inquiry that most accurately captures my approach to medicine and my investigation of stem cells.

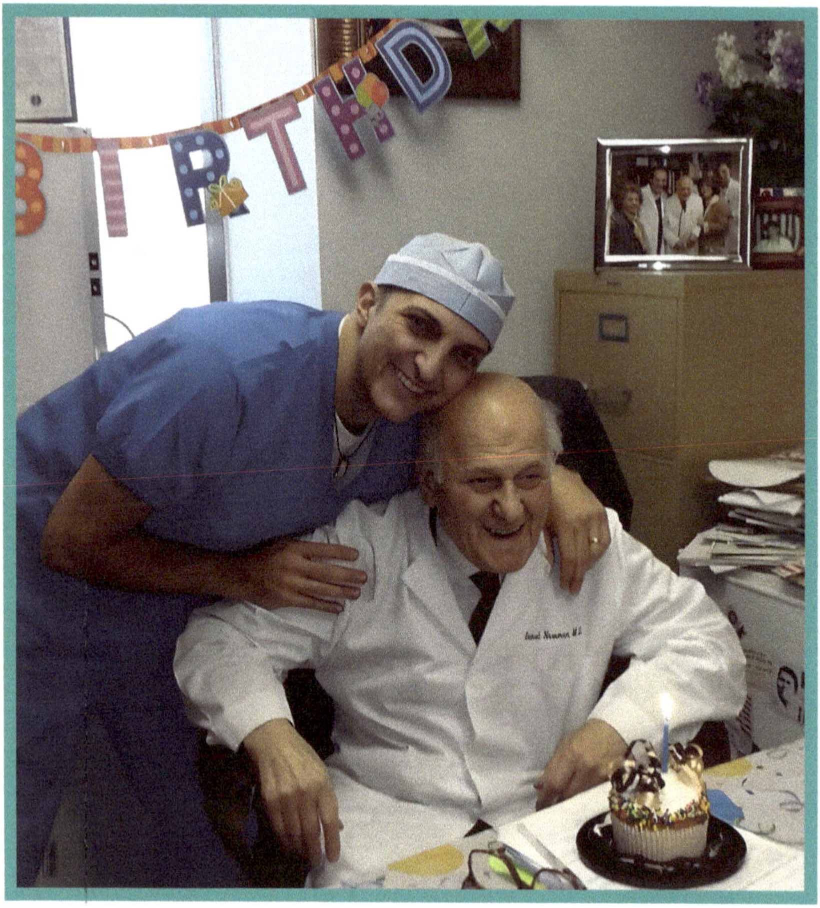

My father and me

In the early 2000s, clinicians and researchers had begun to make breakthroughs in their understanding of the nature of fat cells, the makeup of adipose tissue, and in particular, the stroma, the connective tissue that holds the cells together. They had discovered that within the stroma was a reservoir of adult mesenchymal stem cells or adipose-derived stem cells (ASCs) that can divide indefinitely and are capable of differentiating and producing various tissues, such as fat, bone, and cartilage. This meant that these stem cells could regenerate our tissues.

Still in my training, I was actively investigating this closed system of fat harvesting, wanting to understand how to most effectively utilize it for dermatologic, reconstructive, and cosmetic purposes. I focused on the components of the fat tissue itself and observed that, once removed into the syringe, it would separate into different layers: the top layer made up of oil released from damaged cells during the fat removal, the second layer composed of mature fat cells, and the bottom layer made up of saline and blood. Most notable for me was the discovery that the stem cells were concentrated in the layer *between* the fat cells and the liquid.

Soon into my dermatology and cosmetic practice, I began to work with stem cells, continuing to think about the significance of stem cells existing *between* the layers of fat cells. I also kept returning to the problems and lack of stellar results from the available methods of fat grafting.

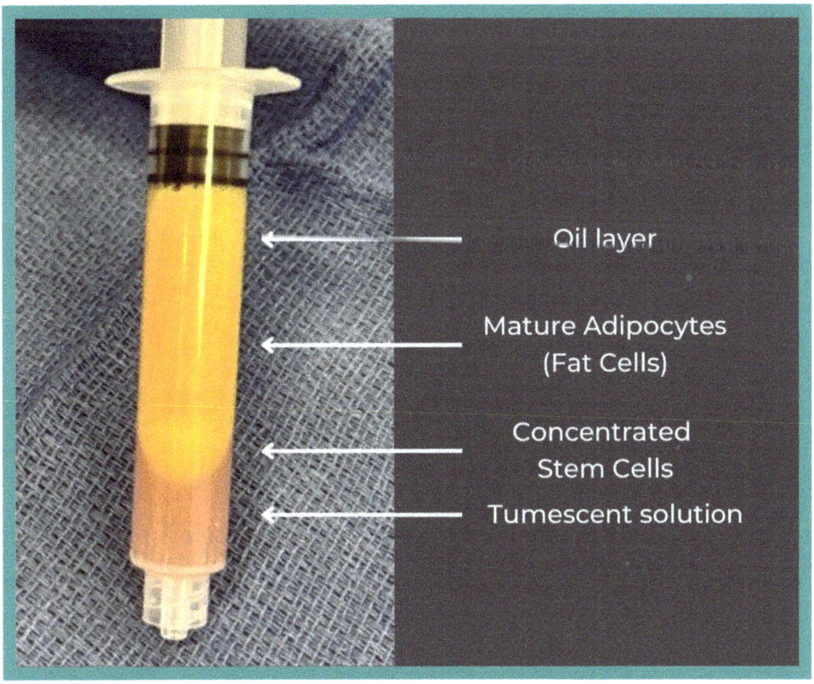

The harvested fat layers in a syringe

The Differences Between Fat Transfer, Fat Grafting, and Fat Injection

Fat transfer Taking fat from one part of the body and placing it in another part of the body. It can be a chunk of fat or isolated fat cells.

Fat grafting Introducing fat into a new location on the body and incorporating and attaching that live fat into the new area with new blood vessels and other support structures that it needs to survive and function.

Fat injection Injecting isolated fat cells through a hollow needle or cannula (a blunt-tipped hollow needle).

Most doctors were using fat grafting as a technique to simply fill hollows and folds on the face (such as laugh lines to try to make patients look younger) or to try to correct disfigurements, such as an indentation on the breast after cancer surgery. But I had the distinct feeling that we were missing something.

The Eureka Moment

At the time, most physicians were using techniques that overlooked the vital reservoir of adult stem cells within the fat. In the open system, the rich stem cells in the liquid were unknowingly washed away in the sieve, along with oils and blood, and then discarded. Stem cells were never part of the consideration in the open method; the focus was exclusively on the fat itself. However, in the new closed system method, the released stem cells between the fat cells could be preserved within the syringe into which the fat was being suctioned.

I have dedicated myself to always looking to learn more and seek out better, more effective approaches to healing. It is this spirit of inquiry that most accurately captures my approach to medicine and my investigation of stem cells.

I studied the most up-to-date research at the time and then did some of my own investigating, ultimately hypothesizing that it wasn't the fat cells that were producing the rejuvenating effects, but the stem cells between them. I also focused on the fact that regenerative cells make up 2 to 10 percent of fat tissue, which reinforced the benefit of using fat as the preferred tissue from which to harvest the autologous stem cells—clearly the fat tissue is the richest in stem cells out of all tissues in the body.

I was certain that the reason I began to see better results using the closed syringe method was because the closed system preserved the stem cells. But despite the closed system improving results and reducing complications, the overall clinical outcomes were still unpredictable. In most cases, only 20 to 50 percent of the volume of fat that was successfully grafted onto a patient would become part of the tissue. I wanted better and more predictable results. In my quest to develop and optimize the fat grafting system, through ongoing clinical and laboratory procedures and practices, I was discovering and coming to a pivotal conclusion: when this liquid was being discarded, so were the potent stem cells. This was an aha moment as I realized that the reason why the closed system was yielding superior results to the open system was precisely because in the open system, the stem cells in the fat were being discarded, whereas they were preserved with the closed system. I kept thinking about the importance of the fact that stem cells are harbored in fat and how utilizing fat as part of the substrate increased its healing power. I wanted to understand how to best preserve these stem cells and reuse them instead of discarding them. This realization was a turning point in my mission to advance the field of stem cell therapy in its infancy so that it was wholly reliable, predictable, and used to its vast potential for self-healing.

Discovering the potential of the naturally rich and concentrated stem cells layer within the fat I was harvesting from my patients motivated me to further explore how I could potentially improve the results of the reinjection of the stem cells even more. Another important consideration was the environment in which the cells existed. I knew that the quality of the cells was affected by environment—not only the rich liquid in which the stem cells reside but also the graft into which they're being introduced. This realization set me on a totally new path to improve the whole process from fat removal to fat injection.

As I advanced through my fellowship training in cosmetic surgery, I continued to learn and improve the closed method harvesting procedure. The most commonly used method of fat removal at the time was liposuction, which had become relatively easy and safe to perform. This method was very aggressive in its use of a long hollow tube (called a *cannula*) with grater-like, sharp-edged holes along its tip, and the excessive power used by the suction machine to remove or inject the fat severely damaged the fat cells during the harvesting process. Along with new publicized scientific discoveries, each treatment helped me to gain more knowledge and improve the fat removal technique to optimize the quality of the cells that would be injected back into the patient in my surgery center. I adjusted the suction level and changed the cannula with sharp-edged holes to one that was blunt-edged to yield the best quality of cells. In addition, I improved both the cannula for injecting the autologous cells back into the patient as well as the injection method, shifting from a bolus of cells into one spot to a layered and precise micro injection of cells.

The next logical hypothesis was to separate the stem cells from the other components and then concentrate them before reinjecting them. Initially, the idea of concentrating the stem cells was to improve the percentage of the graft "take" and the predictability of the results. If we were getting better results with the simple syringe method, how much better would it be if we increased the ratio of the stem cells to the fat cells? Again, I knew it wasn't just the fat that was making a difference in these procedures; it was the stem cells within the fat. I was hypothesizing that there must be a way to facilitate or perhaps direct how stem cells regenerate tissues in the body, and I was determined to utilize this understanding in order to find a method to help the body to do what it knows best: naturally heal itself.

My Approach to Healing

The more I delved into the promise and potential of stem cell therapy, the more my approach to medicine and treatment began to shift. Although I'm trained as a dermatologist and a cosmetic surgeon, as a physician I see the whole person and I strive to help every person in need in any condition, whether by treating them myself, by providing advice, or by referring them to my colleagues. I am committed to finding the best and most advanced medical care for my patients.

I understood the science of stem cells, I appreciated the body's natural intelligence to heal itself, and I followed its pathways. I didn't interfere with or manipulate the process. I observed it, studied it, and then developed a technology to imitate it, staying as close to nature as possible. What is clear through my own research and that of many other esteemed scientists who have come before me is that when we give the body what it needs, it can continue working optimally. When utilized properly, stem cells help us redefine aging, support longevity, and enable radiance from within. Stem cells offer us a way to retain our functioning, improve our well-being, and enhance our quality of life—naturally so—instead of thinking about aging as an inevitable loss of vitality.

The fact that the underlying mechanisms that make stem cells so powerful apply to all aspects of physiology empowered me to help many different types of patients heal from all sorts of conditions. But perhaps even more importantly, this made me realize that stem cell technology had the potential to reframe the way we thought about aging and disease altogether, which led me to explore how stem cell technology could not only prevent disease but optimize functioning in many other ways. Rather than wait to treat illness or disease states, I wanted to harness the regenerative power of the body and learn how to tap into its own innate drive to renew and protect itself from environmental insults and the impacts of daily living by providing protective and preemptive measures.

Rather than wait to treat illness or disease states, I wanted to harness the regenerative power of the body and learn how to tap into its own innate drive to renew and protect itself from environmental insults and the impacts of daily living by providing protective and preemptive measures.

My particular, holistic approach to stem cell therapy offers a new way to think about the aging process. Stem cells give people an opportunity to reconsider their own situations and imagine lives beyond chronic disease and the supposed inevitable loss of functioning that accompanies getting older. This outlook is the basis of regenerative medicine and my belief that aging is not a disease, but rather a natural part of living. In the cycle of life, there is always a beginning and an end. Aging, at the cellular level, is simply a slowing down of the body's systems because the body's cells—from neurons to skin to muscles and bones—become less efficient at their jobs. Aging means that tissues that break down are not replaced with the same number of new tissues or at the same rate. Tissues need more time to recover, and the immune system has to work harder to protect against and/or fight disease and illness. Within this lens, aging is not something to fear or fight against but to understand and ideally manage better so we can slow and delay the ill effects that happen with aging while also enjoying a better quality of life.

Aging is not something to fear or fight against but to understand and ideally manage better so we can slow and delay the ill effects that happen with aging while also enjoying a better quality of life.

I also believe strongly that people will do a much better job at preserving the healthy functioning of their brains and bodies if they grow a keener appreciation for how our bodies work. When you understand more about how and why the body functions as it does, you become more aware of what to do to improve your overall health and appearance. You are empowered with the proper information on how to take charge of your health and well-being and make responsible and educated decisions, in support of your optimal living.

Don't you want to be empowered to be your best self at every age?

Are you interested in or motivated to harness the power of creation?

It all comes down to how cells work, especially stem cells.

The promise and hope of advancements in stem cell science are still unfolding, with very encouraging indications for major medical breakthroughs in the near future.

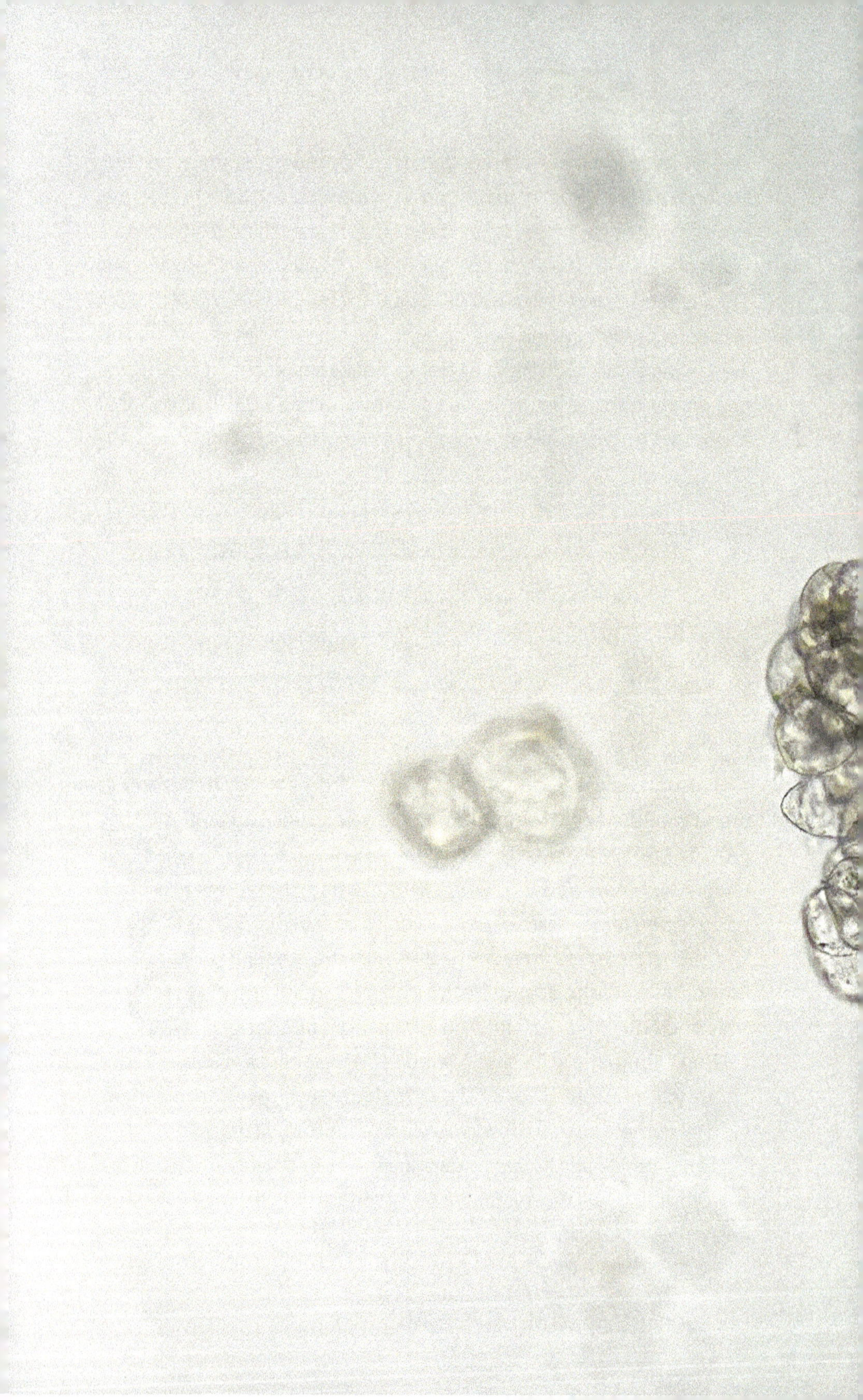

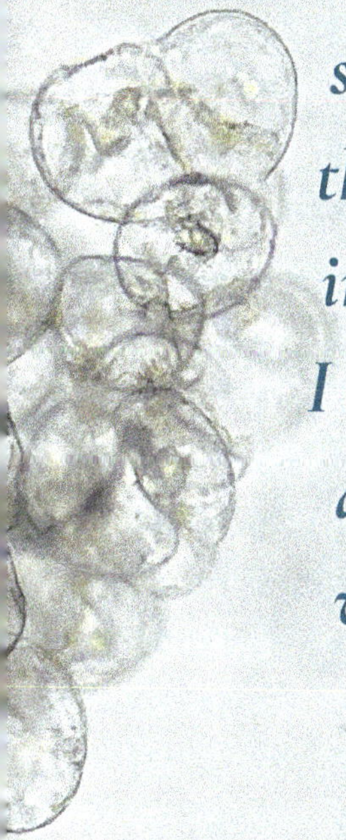

“As much as I use the most innovative and cutting-edge technology in my practice, I still feel in many ways like the “village doctor.” Following in my father’s footsteps, I care for my patients deeply and strive to provide them with the best care possible.”

—DR. NATHAN NEWMAN

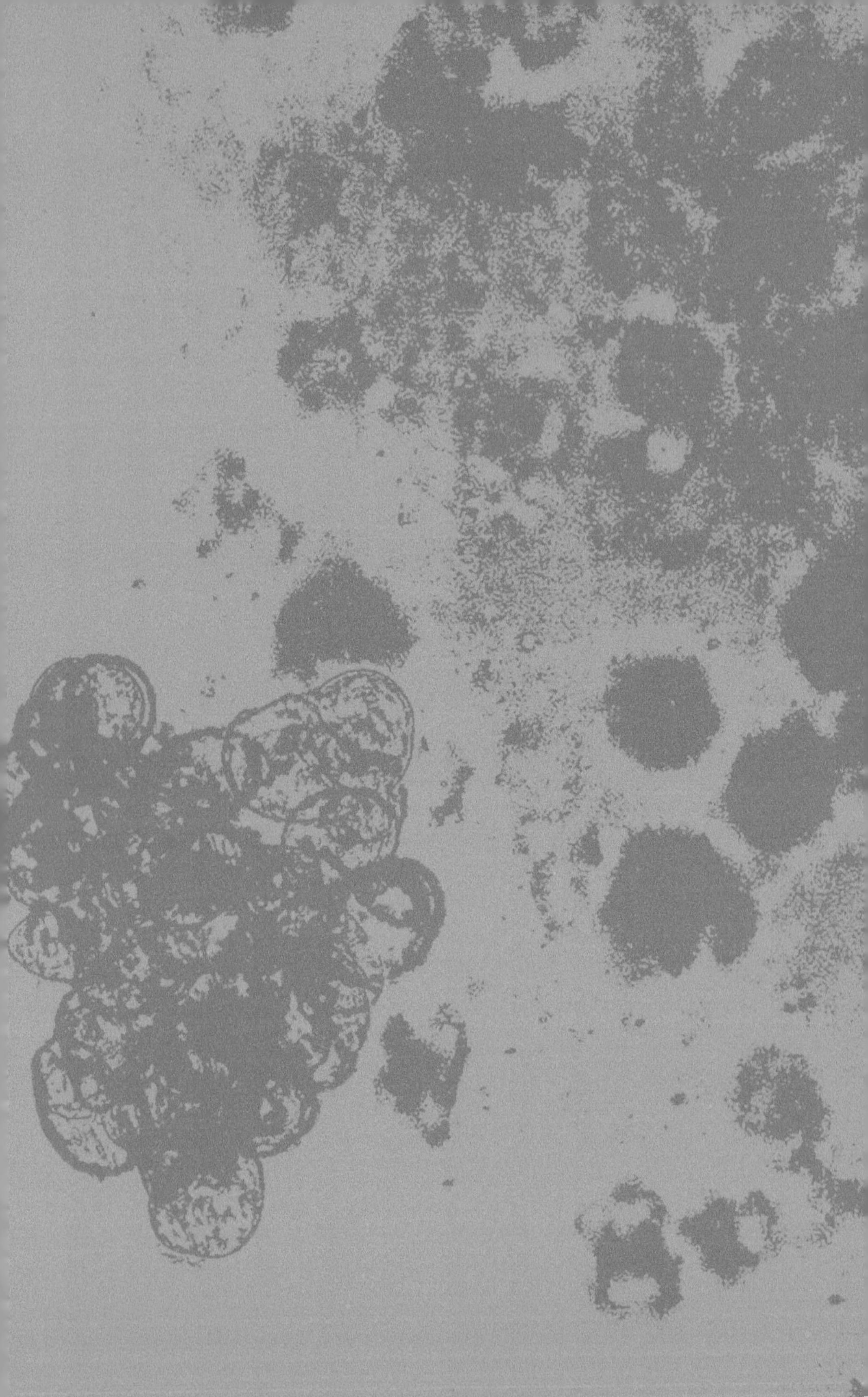

2

Where It All Began

In many ways, this book has been in my heart for more than 25 years—ever since I first opened the doors to my private surgical center and medical practice in Beverly Hills. It's the culmination of a lifelong passion for healing, driven by the belief that every person deserves not just to be treated, but to be truly cared for, with all the compassion and expertise I can offer. This book is a testament to that commitment, and to the belief that true healing is about more than just treating a condition—it's about providing wholesome and multidimensional therapy to the entire person and transforming lives.

My Stem Cell Story

When I was a little boy, I loved to watch my father work. He was a family doctor who treated everyone and every condition that he came across in the provincial capital of Hamedan in the northwestern part of Persia. As a generalist, in a time when medical specialties did not exist, he treated ailments from the common cold to gastritis and even delivered babies. He was a true Renaissance man, not just because he spoke eight or nine languages, but also because his approach to medicine was truly holistic: he wanted to help cure the conditions of his patients while also giving them advice on how to eat well, get rest, and energize the body through physical exercise. I think of him now as similar to Maimonides, the great rabbi, philosopher, and physician who also taught his patients about the benefits of living a healthy lifestyle, while addressing all aspects of the human being—physical, emotional, and spiritual. Like him, I have always known that understanding how these three dimensions of our life are connected and feed off each other is the only way to treat a person as a whole.

Back in Persia, my father was the gynecologist, the internal medicine doc, and even the coroner. He did everything for everyone—from people in the upper echelon of the community and those who could

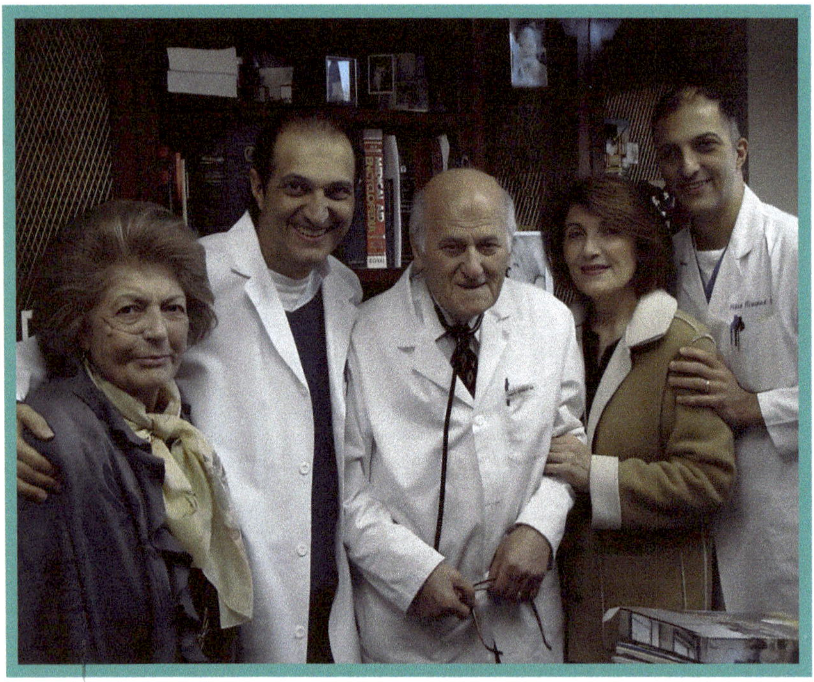

My parents, siblings, and me

only pay him with a chicken, yogurt, or a batch of spring vegetables. People gathered in front of his office, often forming a line around the block, seeking healing and comfort. I vividly remember sitting on my father's lap in his clinic at the tender age of six, watching the diverse group of patients who walked daily through the heavy wooden doors of the three-story building. One day as I was observing my father's work, he approached a patient who was lying on the examination table and put a needle in the patient's stomach, setting off a spouting surge of yellow fluid. The spurt of liquid fascinated me, but more amazing than that in my child's eyes was the patient's obvious and immediate relief from pain. This and similar instances of witnessing my father heal the sick and injured were transformative, instilling in me a passionate desire to follow in my father's footsteps and carry on his mission of healing, saving, and improving lives through medicine.

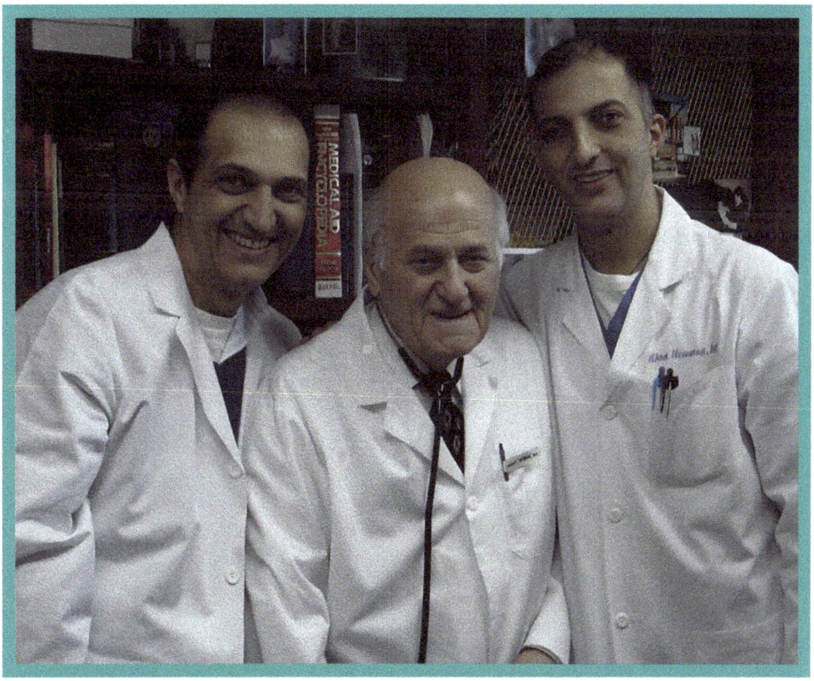

Me with my father, Dr. Samuel Newman, and brother, Dr. Armand Newman

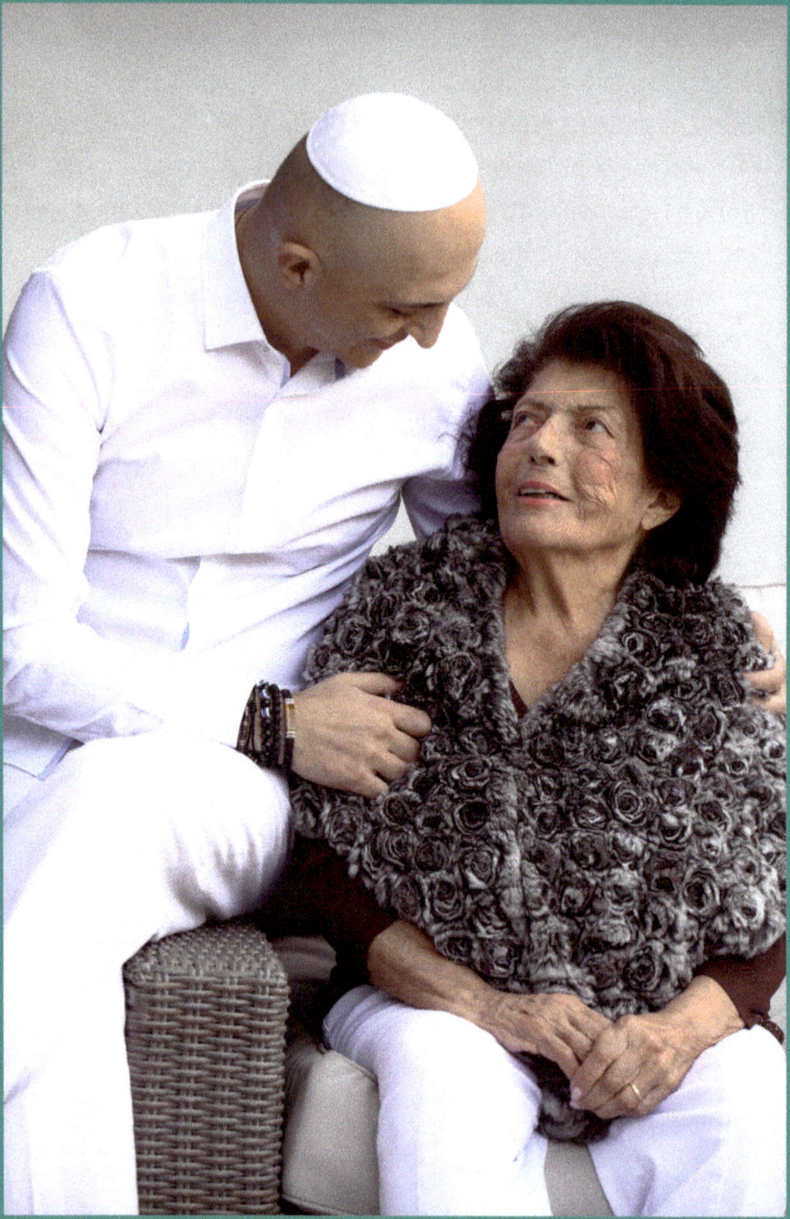

"I am who I am thanks to the love and support of my parents. My mother's natural intelligence, wise guidance, and strong and independent leadership are the key to my personal and professional success and happiness. But most of all, her qualities, her unconditional love and warmth, are and will always be the wind beneath my wings."

—DR. NATHAN NEWMAN

Later when our family emigrated to the US during the Islamic Revolution of 1979, my father had to redo his training and learn English. He'd done his previous medical studies in French. Now he was 50 years old and had to do his training all over again. He was accepted into a competitive medical residency program in family practice at Chicago's Ravenswood Hospital, which was itself an incredible feat for someone of his age and background. At the same time, my older brother was accepted to his medical residency in dermatology in Chicago, so incredibly my father and brother were in residency training at the same time. When their training was complete, our family moved to Los Angeles and my father and brother opened their practice together. I was still in high school, champing at the bit to get started and have the privilege to join them soon.

My father and brother were not the only physicians in our family—my grandparents were also doctors, and my uncles also worked in the medical field as pharmacists, all as intrigued as I was about scientific research. Inspired by this lineage, I pursued medicine even as an undergraduate at the University of Southern California. I engaged in research, investigating the effectiveness of the first sunscreens against skin-damaging UVA rays at the University of California Los Angeles. I also researched the novel anti-aging effects of glycolic acid on the skin, presenting the findings at the American Society for Dermatologic Surgery Meeting in 1992 and publishing them in a medical journal.

During medical school at the Albert Einstein College of Medicine in New York, I continued doing research and also had the opportunity to observe my older brother's dermatology practice. Deeply influenced by my brother's personal mentorship, I then decided that I, too, should become a dermatologist. I returned to Los Angeles briefly to fulfill my internal medicine year at UCLA-Wadsworth VA Hospital and then, following in my father's and brother's footsteps, headed to Chicago to do my residency in dermatology at Cook County Hospital. During my residency, I developed a keen interest in cosmetic surgery and decided to augment my training as a fellow in cosmetic surgery through the American Academy of Cosmetic Surgery in Southern California.

After concluding my 13 years of higher education, I came back to Beverly Hills and opened my clinic and surgery center, next door to my father's and brother's practices. A few years later, I opened my state-of-the-art stem cell research and development facility in Los Angeles County so that I could expand my mission to bring stem cell therapy beyond the clinic and the surgery room. In the past few years, my nephew and two nieces have also completed their surgical and medical training and joined our medical family legacy by becoming physicians.

I feel blessed every day that I get to do what I love, and I'm passionate about continuing my father's legacy as the village doctor. I often feel that more than I was looking for stem cells, *they* found *me*, and now it is my calling and responsibility to share with you the fascinating knowledge I've gained along the way.

More than I was looking for stem cells, *they* found *me*, and now it is my calling and responsibility to share with you the fascinating knowledge I've gained along the way.

The Ability of Stem Cells to Naturally Heal the Body

In the late 1990s, as I was finishing my dermatology residency and cosmetic surgery fellowship, I became fascinated by a then-nascent area of medicine—stem cell therapy. Stem cells are the only cells in our body that can differentiate and transform into a specific cell and become a part of the tissue that surrounds it. For instance, if stem cells are injected into muscle tissue, they turn into muscle cells; if they are introduced into bone, they turn into bone tissue. This unique capacity is what gives stem cells the power to rejuvenate and promote healing to damaged tissues. They can also improve blood flow for faster healing, restore skin integrity due to aging or injury, fill in the hollows below the eyes, mitigate the darkness of the under-eye tissue, and even reverse the sagging that occurs as a face ages. Stem cells are also unique in that they work with the body's own natural intelligence. Indeed, the remarkable potency of stem cells comes from their special ability to differentiate and "speak" to other important cells, tapping into the body's self-healing capacities and directing it to literally *heal itself*.

I have spent the last two decades investigating the enormous potential of stem cells to transform people's health and improve their quality of life. I've helped thousands of my patients recover from trauma, put autoimmune disorders into remission, reverse arthritis, quicken healing from injuries and burns, and rejuvenate their appearance. While most physicians focus on treating patients in the clinic and researchers traditionally conduct their investigations in the lab, I have always approached patient care as a virtuous circle, putting research at the forefront of how I treat patients so that I can give them the most up-to-date, personalized care possible. In medicine, there is a disconnect and lack of understanding of what happens in the clinic and what happens in the lab. Most labs research an area and then try to establish what their findings can do, which may or may not translate easily to clinical practice for the benefit of patients. By connecting my research to clinical practice, I can be more precise, efficient, effective, and comprehensive as I develop solutions that can be used to treat patients in the clinic. This ongoing flow of information allows me to develop, improve, and optimize therapy protocols and product developments accurately and relatively quickly.

Whether patients come to me to restore their appearance and offset aging or to address serious medical conditions due to disease or serious, life-threatening injuries, I always consider the entire cycle of healing—from the clinic to the lab and back again to the clinic. This clinic-to-research-to-clinic method has enabled me to invent and apply a unique stem cell technology to create optimal outcomes, enabling people to heal faster and more fully.

Over 25 years ago, I developed a minimally invasive surgical technique, the Stem Cell Lift, which maximizes the impact of stem cell therapy by using a proprietary process for harvesting and concentrating the rich stem cells from the patient's fat and then reintroducing them to regenerate tissue, enhance healing, and rejuvenate their appearance. I've been utilizing stem cells in this special way to fix disfigurements in the face or body that result from cancer treatments or injury or other conditions where reconstruction is needed. When I perform the Stem Cell Lift for cosmetic patients, who prefer it to the more dangerous traditional facelift, I am able to achieve much more natural results, helping women and men regain their youthful appearance by restoring and enhancing their facial volume, improving their skin's elasticity and texture, and recontouring facial structure to return it to its former proportions.

Understanding that the outcomes I was witnessing at the clinic were not the result of the stem cells themselves, but rather of something the stem cells were producing, inspired me to further research this process. From the scientific research I led with my team of scientists, I learned that the healing and rejuvenating power of stem cells comes from what they secrete and how these secretory factors communicate with their surroundings. This communication is the universal language of all cells—and the basis of my natural intelligence paradigm of stem cells.

My desire to deepen my understanding of this communication and find ways to utilize the stem cells' natural intelligence prompted me to research, develop, and manufacture stem cell products for medicinal and cosmetic use. For instance, my research team and I have created several stem cell–based products derived from human or plant cells that are safe and effective to treat a growing array of conditions, allowing me to share the benefit of my approach to stem cell technology with millions of people from all around the world, who cannot visit me in my California medical center.

The Natural Intelligence of Stem Cells is the culmination of my work as a pioneering expert in developing innovative methods for harnessing the power of stem cells to regenerate the body, optimize healing, and rejuvenate appearance. In the pages ahead, I will share my journey, charting the research process that has empowered tens of thousands of people around the globe to take charge of their health, regain function, restore their youthful appearance, and lift their spirits—that's the "lift" inherent in my Stem Cell Lift procedure!

I will also share other key aspects of my work—what I call my *acellular* therapy options—which include innovative methods for directing stem cells. I have led an interdisciplinary team of medical doctors and PhD research scientists specializing in stem cell research to develop a patented biotechnological process that harvests and utilizes both human and plant stem cells, which has allowed us to pioneer new applications of stem cell research. By using a complex, personalized approach to culture and combine cells, we can achieve unique profiles of secretory factors that enable individuals to access off-the-shelf treatments or cosmetics that are safe and effective for them. This breakthrough has opened the door to regenerative medicine for consumers, and we are already seeing incredible results in thousands of women and men who have benefited from this stem cell–based technology. These advancements are now being incorporated into new cosmetic and wellness products available through my biotech company.

I respect and acknowledge the fact that there are many mechanisms and processes that scientists can't fully understand, explain, or prove. It was exactly this assumption that led me to several breakthroughs in how to optimize stem cell therapy and create a wholly original technology to maximize healing results. But I also believe in the human body's innate intelligence—and I don't think we know the half of it!

I was raised by a mother and a father who always valued education and self-advocacy as paramount. As a father and a physician myself, I am driven to do my best to empower society with knowledge and raise awareness about advanced technology and healing methods. The more we understand about how our bodies work, the more motivated and capable we are at making decisions that maintain our health, prevent illness and disease, and help us look and feel our best—regardless of our age. Stem cell technology—both your own and that from plants—can prevent disease conditions, reset your biological clock to slow the momentum of aging, reduce pain, and help you heal faster and more fully from injuries, chronic disease, or autoimmune disorders that you may suffer from. It is my hope that when you appreciate the science behind stem cells that I describe in the pages ahead, you will feel a new sense of hope and motivation to seek out stem cell therapies that are now available to you.

My approach to stem cell technology can halt disease, speed up healing, and slow down the momentum and side effects of aging. In this book, you'll learn the secrets to improving the overall quality of your life so that you and your loved ones can enjoy more years of optimal functioning and joy.

So, before we begin, let me ask you some questions:

- Would you like to live a pain-free life, one that is not restricted by achy or stiff joints?
- Would you like to refresh the way you look, not by over-tightening or plumping up your skin, but by restoring the way you naturally looked in your prime?
- Would you like to reverse inflammatory conditions that make you more vulnerable to illness and trigger disease?
- Would you like to ameliorate healing from an injury?

My approach to stem cell therapy provides you with solutions for these problems and more. Now let's get started.

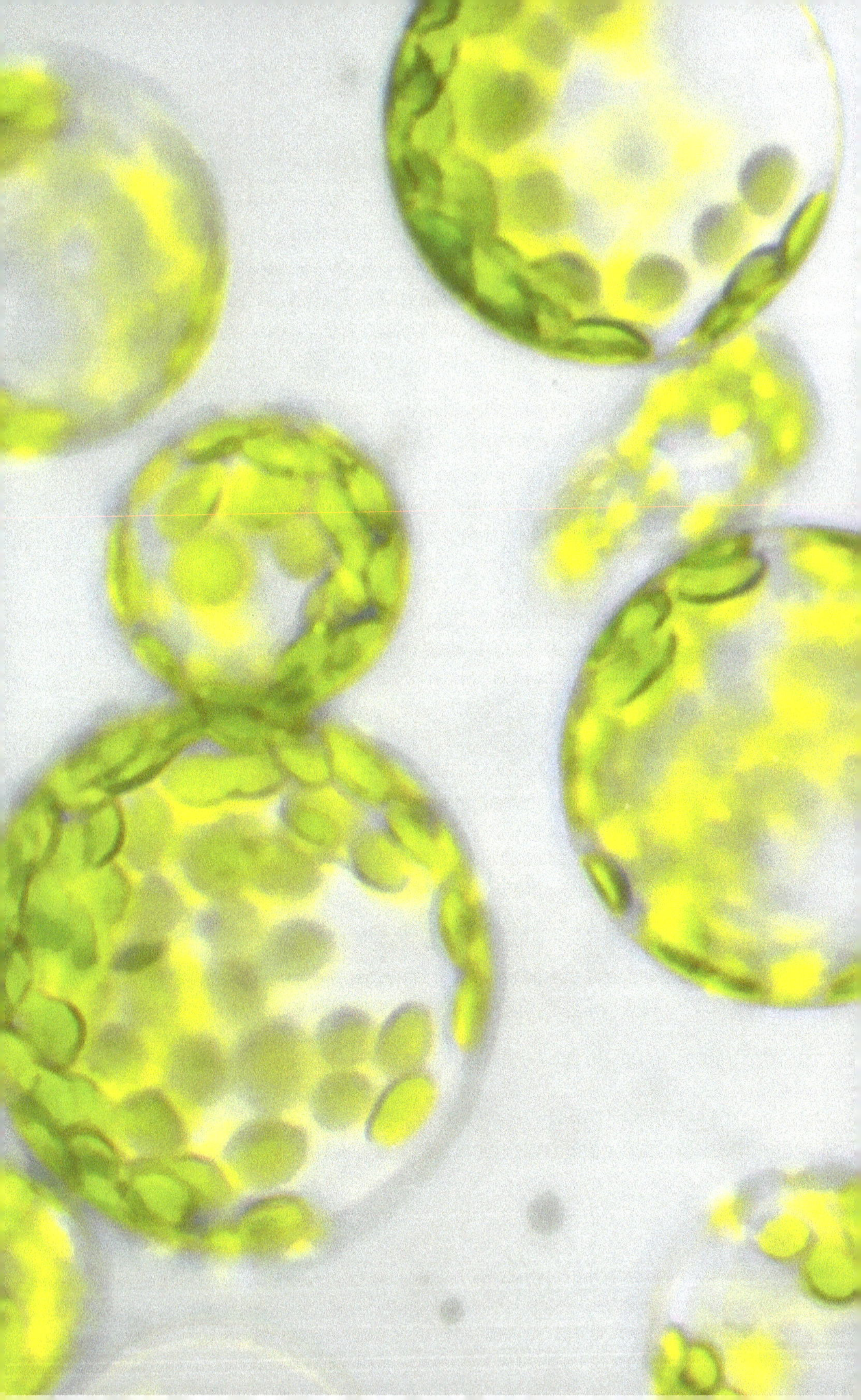

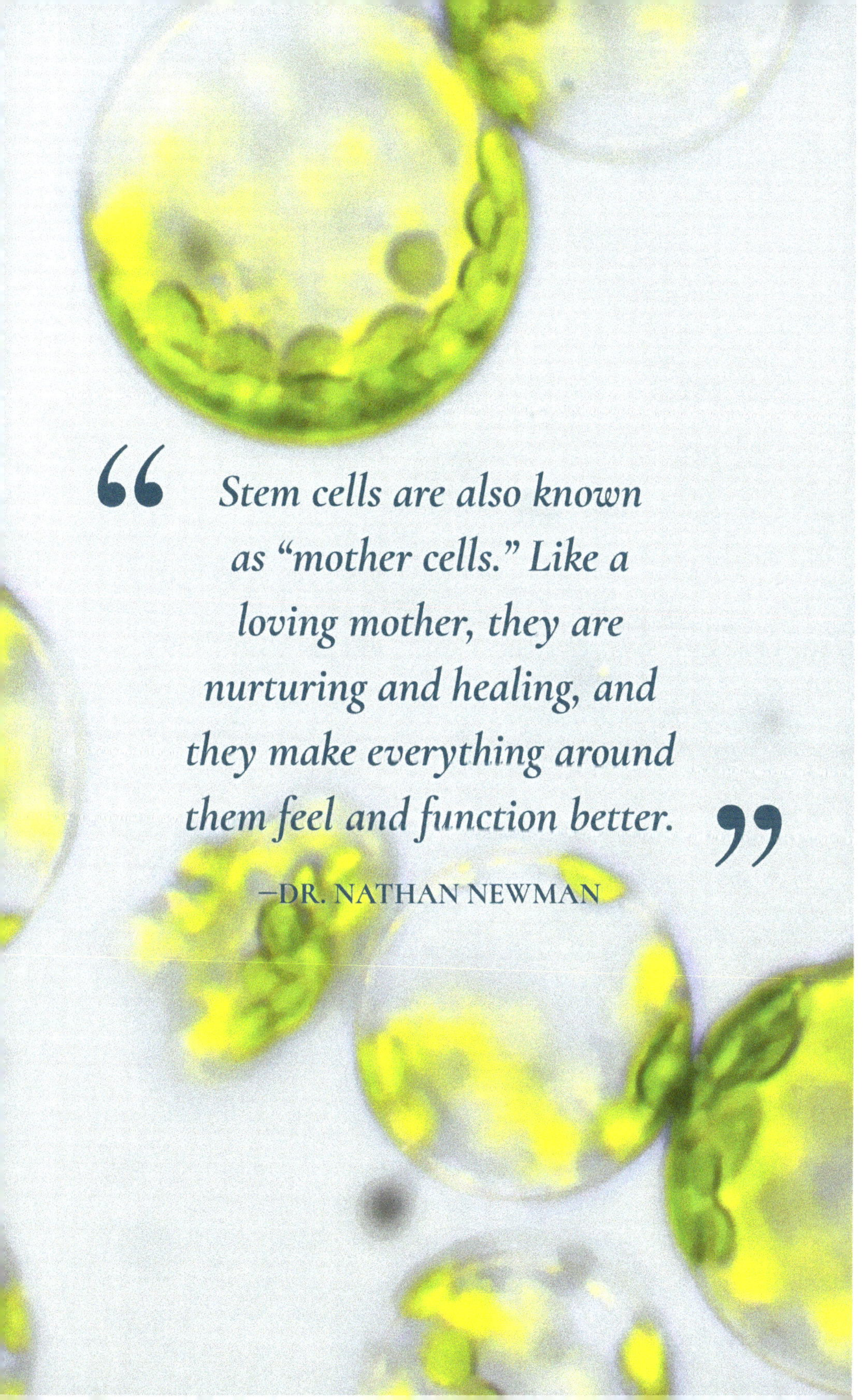

> *Stem cells are also known as "mother cells." Like a loving mother, they are nurturing and healing, and they make everything around them feel and function better.*
>
> —DR. NATHAN NEWMAN

3

Inventing the Stem Cell Lift Method

As soon as I had set up my clinical practice and surgery center in Beverly Hills, I knew I wanted to continue to follow the threads of research that I had been investigating when I was first experimenting with fat grafting in Chicago and later during my fellowship in cosmetic surgery. Knowing that of all the tissues in the body, fat contained the highest density of stem cells, I began to test different methods of separating the stem cells from the fat and concentrating them in order to optimize clinical results. I also began to investigate the nuances of how to optimally use human stem cells to promote healing, regenerate the body and face, and improve longevity and quality of life.

Before this time, the scientific belief was that we are born with and die with a set number of cells in our brains and many parts of the body, including the fat cells, and that these cells don't generally change in number, get replaced, or can regenerate. There was less understanding about where stem cells were located or even their function. Over the past 25 years, our collective knowledge about the power of stem cells has grown exponentially. We now know, for instance, that these powerful cell types exist in almost all the tissues of the body. As mentioned, one of the first ways that stem cells were used was through bone marrow transplantation to treat blood-borne cancers, but it has taken years to truly understand and appreciate the potential for stem cells to bring all levels of healing through the lens of regenerative medicine.

As I continued to grow my therapeutic uses of stem cell science, I was getting very good results for my cosmetic and dermatologic patients who were coming to me to address the common effects of aging—sagging skin, loose jowls, wrinkles around the eyes and mouth, and other such issues. My practice was growing with each year, and I should have been satisfied, but I knew there was something more I could be achieving with stem cell technology.

I wanted to perfect my method for both harvesting the autologous stem cells and concentrating them to create a more robust, effective response when they were reintroduced. I felt strongly that there was a more exact, directed way to produce optimal results. Up until this point, stem cells were not used in such a personalized manner, and fat grafting often created unwanted outcomes or less-than-permanent results. In my dermatology and cosmetic practice, it became my professional mission to invent a novel procedure that maximized the use of stem cells derived from a patient's own fat.

I had been systemizing the manner in which I extracted my patients' stem cells from their fat tissue, then separating the stem cells from the surrounding stoma between the fat cells, and then creating a concentrated stem cell mixture to inject back into the desired area. My method of both safely extracting the stem cells using the tools that I had designed and then concentrating the stem cells (thereby building their potency) was a differentiator that enabled me to achieve more precise, immediate, and lasting results for my patients.

What did this mean?

I had perfected the ability to put the stem cells where I wanted them to go! If a woman wanted to fill in the hollows around her eyes, my method could reach that exact area. If a man wanted to reduce the wrinkles on his face or neck, reinjecting a concentrated amount of his autologous stem cells to those areas restored his skin's elasticity and texture. By their very nature, the cells knew exactly what to do: regenerate the tissue that was being lost to aging. But I had the distinct sense that it was not just the fat or the stem cells producing these results; it was the environment surrounding the stem cells that was contributing to their efficacy.

By their very nature, the cells knew exactly what to do: regenerate the tissue that was being lost to aging. But I had the distinct sense that it was not just the fat or the stem cells producing these results; it was the environment surrounding the stem cells that was contributing to their efficacy.

Meet Hersel: The Tipping Point

It was during this time that I received a phone call from a young man named Hersel, who had heard from a friend about my therapeutic work using stem cells. Hersel had suffered from parotid gland cancer, a specific type of tumor affecting the right side of his face and neck. What the surgery had not removed, the radiation had burned, creating an excruciatingly painful scar that went deep into his tissue. He was left with a partially disfigured face and near-constant physical pain. When I met him, his face showed a large sunken hole, with the skin tissue scarred from the radiation. The nerve endings trapped beneath the scar tissue caused tremendous discomfort, and thus far, no doctor had been able to treat him in a way that offered relief. Not only was Hersel suffering physically, but as a young single man, he had become self-conscious, depressed, and withdrawn due to his facial disfigurement.

In his desperate search for help, Hersel had gone to the top hospitals and reconstructive surgeons in hopes of a solution. Because the scars and the radiation had obliterated most of his blood vessels, any attempt to surgically correct or even inject any product to correct the defect would result in loss of blood flow to the skin. Any procedure that other doctors had tried had to be stopped in the middle, because of the poor blood circulation within the thinned scarred skin; any cutting or pressure caused by injection of fillers only caused the skin to die and ulcerate.

In our first meeting, Hersel looked at me with pleading eyes and asked, "Can you fix me?"

I examined him and listened to his story, sensing his anguish and wanting to help. I finally said, "I don't know how much I can help you, but I'm willing to try."

I then explained to Hersel that I couldn't predict how or if I could make any improvement, but I thought that injecting stem cells was his only viable option. I assured him I would do my best to help him in his quest to eliminate his physical and emotional pain and reconstruct the deformity on his face.

Hersel finally had hope that he might achieve a pain-free and functional life, and giving him this ray of hope made me try even harder. Again, I returned to the idea that environment mattered.

Long before we discovered stem cells in the fat, we understood that fat injected next to bone had the capacity to increase the size of the bone. I took some fat from Hersel's flanks and abdomen and decided on a regimen in which I would inject him every three months with his own harvested stem cell–enriched fat into the jaw area. Combining both my dermatological and cosmetic surgery expertise, I wanted to go slowly to see if the stem cells would begin to break down and soften the underlying scar tissue in order to improve his blood flow. At

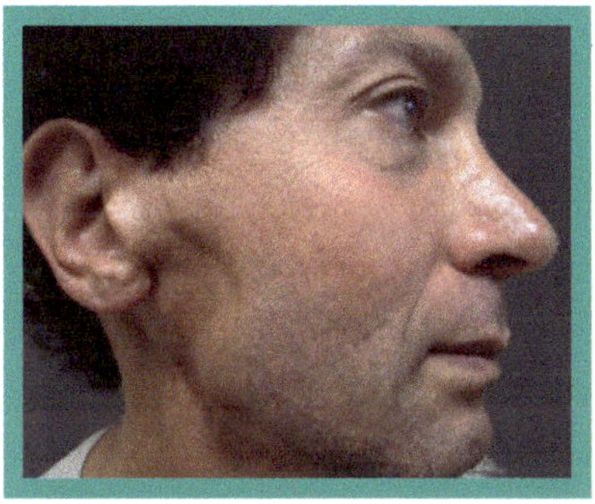

Before

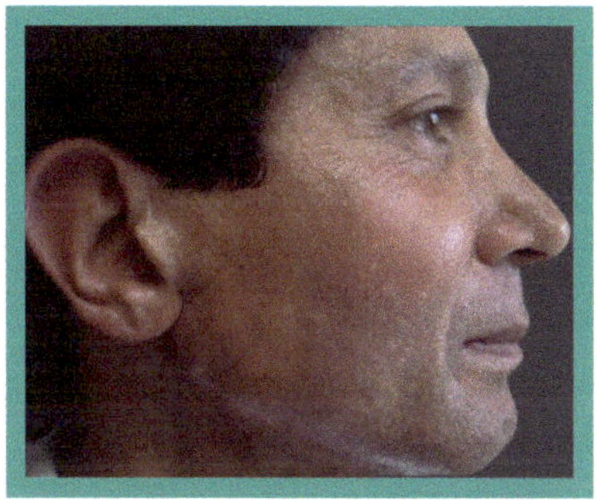

Three years after the first SCL treatment

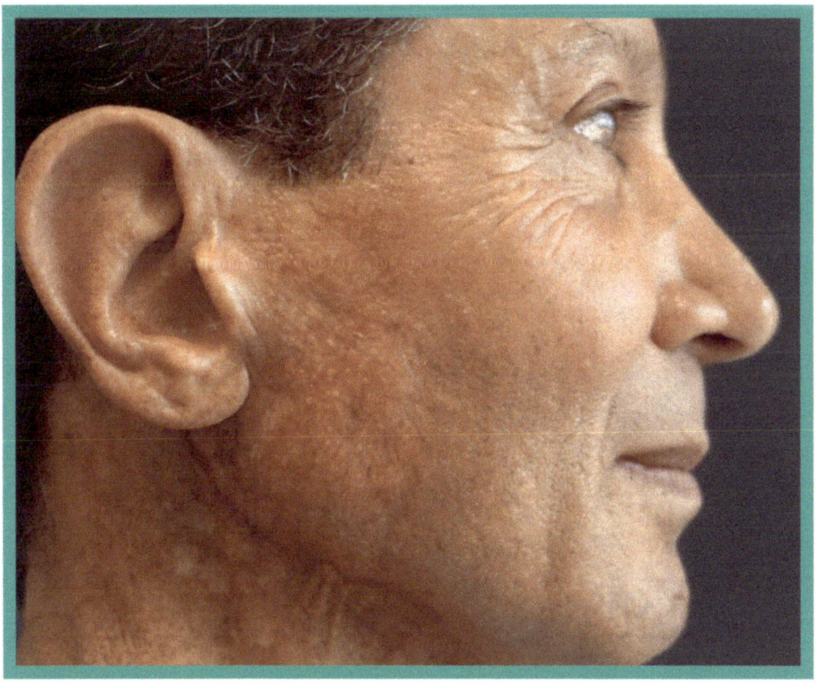

Twelve years after the first SCL treatment

Hersel's life-changing results not only restored his confidence but also eliminated his pain.

first, I injected the cells at the edges of the hardened tissue. My goal was to increase blood flow and start the healing from the outside in.

Three months after the first treatment, Hersel and I were both impressed with the results: there was evidence that the stem cells were working to break up the scar tissue and increase blood flow. This was a very positive sign.

Over the course of the next two years, I continued with this same regimen every three months. And guess what? Hersel's jawline was restored, the radiation burn on his skin had improved, the skin and tissues had become supple and mobile, his pain was resolved, and the hole in his face was corrected—all of which meant his self-image began to heal, too. We were both elated with this progress.

Stem cells "lift" your skin *and* spirit.

In fact, I was simply blown away. The outcome was substantially better than what I could ever have hoped for or imagined.

My success with Hersel spurred me on and was a pivotal moment in my medical career. It also represented the birth of the Stem Cell Lift (SCL) procedure.

I could now see that stem cell therapy could be used to reconstruct bone and tissue in a direct, personalized way. I was fascinated by the capacity of stem cells to heal Hersel's face, jaw, and neck. It's no exaggeration to say that Hersel's life changed because of this stem cell treatment. As he said to me, "You gave me back my life." Hersel had gone from being a young man who believed he could never again have an enjoyable social life to an invigorated person full of hope, energy, and vitality.

My experience with Hersel and what I learned through this clinical application of autologous stem cells deepened my commitment to understanding how best to utilize the science of stem cells to help more people. I wanted to continue to help people look and feel better using stem cell technology for cosmetic purposes, but my experience with Hersel broadened my hopes and made me believe that I had just scratched the surface of their healing potential. I knew that the way in which I retrieved, prepared, and then injected Hersel's stem cells was unique. My method of extracting his fat and stem cells, separating the two types of cells from one another, concentrating the stem cells into a more potent complex, and then reintroducing them had not only accelerated his healing by getting past the scar tissue and breaking it down, but also helped him actually regrow bone and skin tissue. Hersel's results were truly remarkable and a testament to the power of stem cells to regenerate and heal the human body. Hersel was also the ultimate tipping point in clarifying my approach and the SCL procedure, where your own stem cells "lift" your skin *and* spirit.

As you will soon see, I've been privileged to help transform thousands of my patients' lives, using the SCL to address not only cosmetic concerns and signs of aging but also reconstructive (post cancer, musculoskeletal injury, and soft tissue trauma), autoimmune (lichen sclerosus), and musculoskeletal (arthritis, joint pain, and muscle and tendon tears) ailments.

I invented the SCL procedure so that it becomes a gift that keeps on giving. The stem cells repair and rejuvenate, enabling you to feel positive and hopeful now and into the future. The most beautiful part? The SCL is natural, healthy, and safe.

The stem cells repair and rejuvenate, enabling you to feel positive and hopeful now and into the future. The most beautiful part? The SCL is natural, healthy, and safe.

How the Stem Cell Lift Procedure Works

Since my initial work with Hersel, I have been perfecting the SCL procedure so that it is now a state-of-the-art, minimally invasive, two-to-four-hour procedure performed under local anesthesia. I use the SCL to help not only patients like Hersel who will benefit from reconstruction, but also those suffering from inflammatory skin disease, autoimmune disorders, and joint and musculoskeletal conditions. Before I had perfected and named the procedure, I had been using versions of it to address cosmetic concerns related to the negative effects of aging, including skin tone and texture, sagging skin and wrinkles, and loss of facial and neck volume.

The procedure is relatively simple, very safe, and personalized and includes the following steps, a process I review with each patient:

- I help them decide from which area of the body they wish to have fat cells removed, most commonly from the abdomen, flanks (i.e., the "love handles"), or thighs.
- It is an outpatient procedure where they can go home the same day. There is no need for general anesthesia, cutting, scars, or stitches.
- I then inject a tumescent local anesthetic (sterile saltwater mixed with local anesthetic) using a specially designed blunt instrument to numb the fat tissue.
- After a short wait to allow for the local anesthetic medication to work, I remove the fat into a closed system using a mini-liposuction method through specially designed instruments to minimize damage to the collected cells; protect them from the environment and contamination; and minimize risk of infection.

- The stem cells located between the collected fat cells in the closed system are then mechanically dissociated and concentrated. The stem cell to fat ratio is then increased, usually doubled, in the fat cells being prepared for injection into the desired areas. The ratio of cells and the size of the fat cells may be optimized for specific treatment types, including cosmetic (for skin rejuvenation, augmentation, contouring, volumization, and lift), musculoskeletal (for joints, muscles, or tendons), reconstructive (for face, breast, and bone), wound healing, and/or autoimmune skin disease. For instance, if a patient wants to improve their facial appearance by erasing fine lines and wrinkles and returning volume to the cheekbones and lifting the skin of the neck, they will be given local anesthesia in the areas marked for treatment.

- Then I inject the super-charged adult stem cells extracted from the patient's own body fat, along with some fat cells, into the affected tissues targeted for treatment. In Hersel's case, I injected his stem cells into his jaw and face; in patients who want to rejuvenate their appearance, I might inject their own stem cells into the area around their mouth, lips, eyes, or cheeks (see Chapter 8 for specific before and after photos).

- Bandages are placed on the areas where the fat was taken, and small pieces of tape are used to cover the needle marks in the treated areas until the next morning.

- Patients do not require narcotic pain relievers. Ice packs and acetaminophen are all that's needed.

The entire procedure is done all on the same day in less than four hours. Patients are able to walk and resume normal daily activities almost immediately after the SCL procedure. I like to tell my patients that the SCL is like having two procedures at once: the fat harvesting is the bonus—take it from where you don't want it and put it where you need it. My patients love this feature: the SCL can sculpt your face while also sculpting your body.

After the procedure, patients will experience some drainage of the excess saltwater and anesthetic solution from where the fat was removed and may also experience some soreness, similar to what you might expect to feel in your muscles after strenuous exercise. Patients may also feel some tightness or a light throbbing sensation in the injected areas for the first couple of days, which can be readily alleviated with cool compresses and acetaminophen to help reduce swelling and discomfort. Soreness at the fat harvesting site may last about two weeks; however, most patients can resume normal daily routines and exercise immediately, according to their comfort level. Any mild swelling will go away within a few days, though in some rare cases, some patients may experience moderate swelling that can extend for about two weeks after the procedure, especially if bruising occurs. These post-procedure effects are nothing like the bruising, swelling, and pain experienced after traditional facelift surgeries—which is why I refer to SCL as cutting-edge (plastic) surgery without the cutting. (See the section "How the SCL Is Different from Other Procedures" on page 52 to learn how the Stem Cell Lift contrasts with the typical facelift.)

As Amy said after the SCL procedure, "At 39 years old, I had terrible bags under my eyes, making me look tired all the time and much older than my actual age. Dr. Newman performed the Stem Cell Lift on me, and I drove home that day!"

Another patient, Heather said that her biggest concern was resolving the tired look that the dark, thin circles under her eyes were causing. "What you can't see in the pictures is the incredible boost to my self-confidence," she said. "When I get up in the morning, instead of dreading that first glance in the mirror, I get up and actually look forward to seeing my face!"

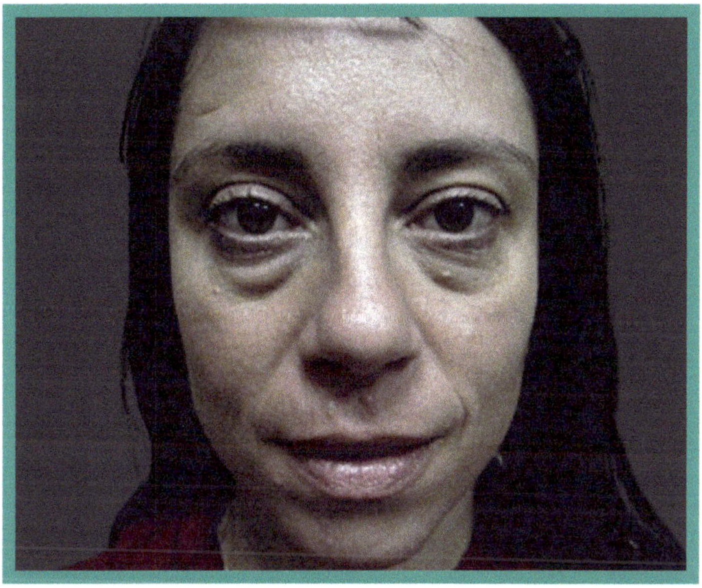

Before

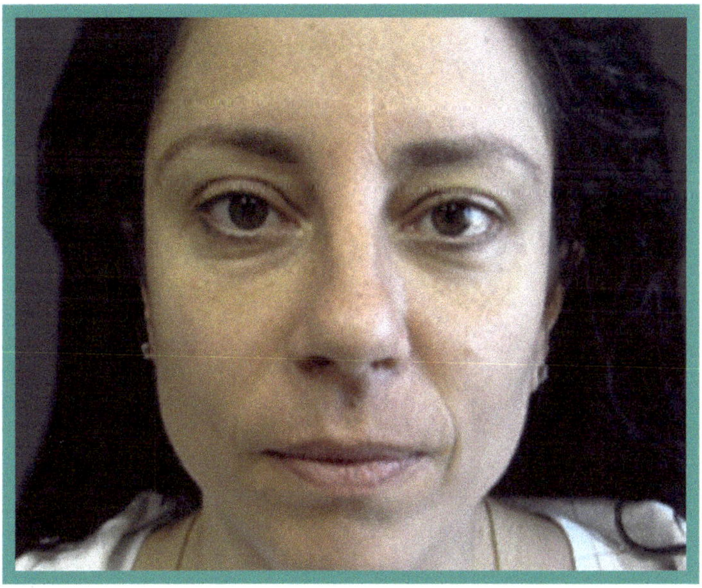

After 1.5 years

Amy's results from the scar-free Stem Cell Lift show how naturally youthful she looks immediately after the procedure to correct her under-eye bags and restore her youthful proportions.

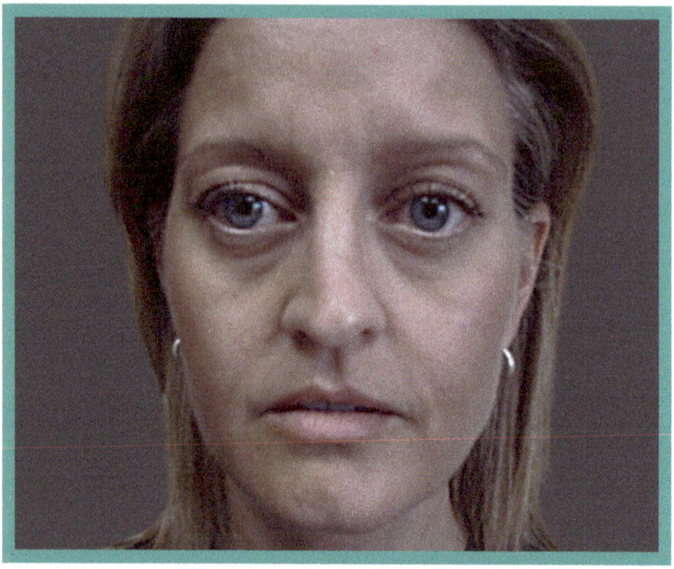

Before

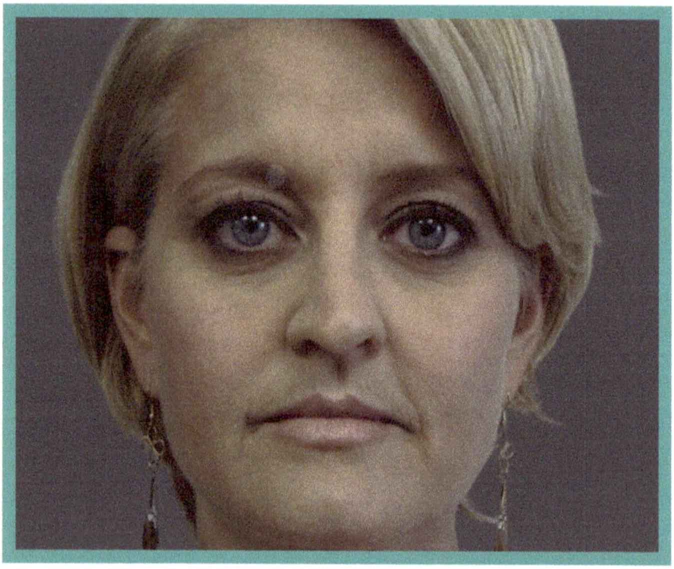

After three years

As an avid runner, Heather was unhappy with the thin, aged, and skeletonized appearance of her face. The results continue to improve. Even three years after her SCL, she is enjoying the long-lasting results.

There are four specific features of the SCL that make it so powerful:

1. The rich concentration of the stem cells that I can gather through the SCL procedure enables the desired regenerative effects on the face and the body.
2. The cells are concentrated into a specific area of the body and exert a focused and robust effect on the targeted tissues.
3. The functional quality of these cells has maintained their regenerative potency.
4. The SCL cell concentration process has activated the stem cells to respond immediately, creating lasting results after three months.

The stem cells will be fully incorporated into the desired tissue about three months after the procedure, after which the results are permanent. Some patients may require additional treatments to maximize the results. Further, some patients may continue to see improvement in the treated areas for up to a year or more, as part of the body's natural healing process. Unlike with traditional cutting and scarring surgeries, where secondary procedures involve more risk and are more difficult to perform, any future SCL procedures are easier to perform and build upon the already grafted stem cells and regenerated scaffolding structures to achieve optimal results.

There are very few if any risks to the SCL. Although rare, in the scientific literature there are reports that some patients have experienced trouble with tissue grafting, occlusion of vessels, uneven skin, lumps under the skin, infection, fat necrosis, scarring, and graft failure—again, these reactions are rare. In my practice of nearly 30 years, I have seen fewer than 10 cases of infection or graft failure.

The Bonus of Adding Platelet-Rich Plasma Treatment

When performing the SCL, I often include another element to maximize the healing effect. By incorporating platelet-rich plasma (PRP), which involves taking blood from a patient (like any routine blood draw) and combining it with stem cells, I am able to accelerate wound healing and tissue grafting. PRP also enhances stem cell activity. The platelets release growth factors that stimulate the stem cells and aid in wound healing, enhancing the results of the SCL procedure by improving cell survival, and boosting regenerative effects.

PRP can be used on its own or in combination with the SCL procedure. While PRP does not provide volume or act as a filler, it serves as a powerful stem cell booster or activator. It can be injected directly into the targeted tissues with a needle or a blunt cannula, and can also be added to stem cells and fat during injection as an enhancer. As you will learn later, PRP acts similarly to the Consortia Factors that improve the overall environment I help to create to maximize results for individual patients. (See the section “The Paracrine Effect” on page 130 for more on PRP and Consortia Factors.)

How the Stem Cell Lift Is Different from Other Procedures

The SCL offers a new, wholly transformative option to help my patients achieve the most natural-looking, permanent results. As a procedure it represents a radical transition from archaic methods with limited results to a new frontier in health, healing, and longevity. Until this technology, surgeons relied on a knife and sutures as their main tool to carry out procedures on their patients. The SCL changes the entire approach to how we can treat our patients. Instead of cutting and moving tissues, we can now use the innate healing power of your stem cells to heal, repair, and rejuvenate tissues. Cutting creates scars, resulting in decreased flexibility, insufficient blood flow, and reduced function of the area. SCL does exactly the opposite: it heals the tissues to restore function while at the same time improving the quality of the tissues by enhancing blood flow and tissue matrix. This changes the entire surgical approach from an invasive and traumatizing experience to a minimally invasive procedure to restore function, enhance youthful facial proportions and symmetry, and improve long-term tissue health. Patients heal in a fraction of the time of traditional surgery with much less risk, pain, complications, and downtime—and no unsightly scars.

Remember Hersel, the patient whose jaw and neck were disfigured after the surgical removal and radiation treatment of a cancerous tumor? When I used my SCL procedure, I used his own adipose stem cells in three-month intervals to signal his innate repair system to break down his scar tissue, generate blood cells, increase blood circulation to the affected region, heal the skin from the radiation burn, and trigger the regrowth of bone and soft tissue—all of which restored full functioning and improved his appearance. For Hersel and many more patients, the use of stem cell therapy has transformed their lives. I hear again and again from my patients how stem cells have brought them renewed confidence and joy and given them a new lease on life—naturally so.

I hear again and again from my patients how stem cells have brought them renewed confidence and joy and given them a new lease on life—naturally so.

PART II

How Stem Cells Repair, Restore, and Rejuvenate

> *“Hearing patient success stories is precisely what inspires me and drives my passion to continue my work on advancing stem cell therapy and technology.”*
>
> —DR. NATHAN NEWMAN

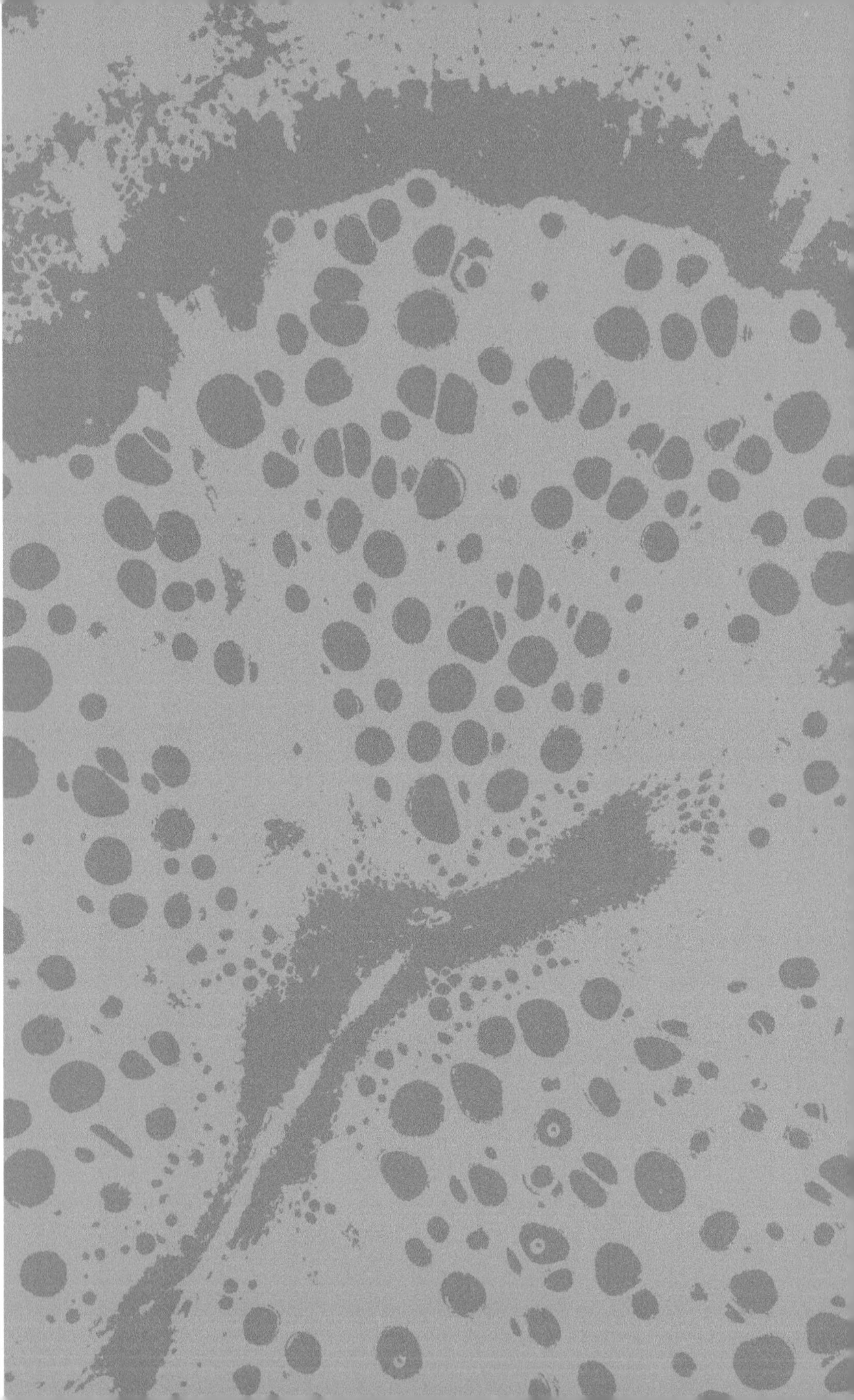

4

How the Stem Cell Lift Builds Back Bone and Tissue

Hersel was my very first patient who benefited from the Stem Cell Lift procedure for purposes of reconstruction—but he became a pivotal patient whose situation pushed me to continue researching the clinical applications of stem cell technology. I knew I was onto something, but I didn't quite realize the immense power and versatility of stem cells.

Meet Jin: Stem Cells Work to Heal Injuries

When I met Jin Jing in May of 2019, she had traveled to my office in Beverly Hills from China in hopes of saving her leg. She was a young mother in a wheelchair who could not stand, much less walk. Two years prior, she had fallen 15 stories from her home balcony and incredibly survived. She told me that she was on the balcony with her father when she tripped and lost her balance. She remembers her father desperately grabbing her hand to keep her from falling, but he could not hold on to her as she fell almost 150 feet below into a construction site onto a heap of sand where a temple was being built.

While Jin Jing miraculously survived, she broke almost all of the bones in her body. After a number of surgeries, she was left with scars on her face that left part of her eyebrow cut off. She also suffered from broken bones, scars, and contractures on her extremities. The doctors put in place pins and plates to align and hold together her broken bones. However, after two years in a wheelchair, she still suffered from pain and was unable to raise her arm to wash her hair or use her left hand to hold things. But most troubling was that the bones in her leg were not healing, despite the fixation plates and numerous large external screws that pierced the skin all along her right leg.

After two years, her doctors had told her there was nothing more they could do for her. She was unable to walk unassisted, her leg and other body parts had ceased to heal, and the doctors believed that amputating her right leg was the only way to help avoid further deterioration. With this prognosis, Jin Jing, a single mom to a beautiful two-and-a-half-year-old, was destined to live out her life in a wheelchair. But Jin Jing did not want to give up. I've always thought that most of her motivation was to be able to walk and do things with her young daughter. So after learning from a friend about my work with stem cell technology and specifically the SCL procedure, she decided to take the courageous step and travel halfway around the world to meet me.

Though I knew that my SCL procedure would reduce Jin Jing's pain and discomfort, I was not at all certain that the damage to her bones and joints could be reversed, but I was willing to try. I began by focusing on her legs, arm, hands, and face. Using her own adipose stem cells and local anesthesia, I injected the tissues and joints in the left elbow, forearm, and hands, where the scarring restricted her ability to move. This restriction of her arms was also causing neuropathic pain that radiated down to her hands. Knowing that I had to avoid all the metal plates and screws holding her bones and joints in the elbow, forearm, and wrist, I first injected her right leg, ankle, and foot with her autologous stem cells and fat. To stabilize the injured leg that was not healing, I targeted the spaces between the shattered bones that were held together with metal plates and screws, penetrating the skin that was red, inflamed, and very sensitive. I also injected the indented area of the right leg where she had lost muscle. Next, I injected the scarred and indented forehead skin to repair the tissues. At the end of the procedure, she went to the hotel to sleep.

For the next few days, we carried out some postoperative treatments—including therapeutic ultrasound, advanced vascular circulation enhancement (AVACEN), a form of microcirculation therapy, and our plant stem cell–based serums—as part of our personalized, comprehensive, and cutting-edge approach to patient care to optimize healing, reduce swelling, and decrease inflammation. Even on the first day after the SCL procedure, Jin Jing was better able to move her upper extremity and experienced less pain. Her face showed immediate signs of improvement, and the skin of her legs was less red and irritated. These were all signs of healing.

Now we had to wait for nature to take its course. I knew that it would take at least two to six months for the bones to fuse and the nerves to restore their functioning. Since her condition had been so severe, it was hard for me to predict how well her leg and other parts of her body would regenerate healthy tissues. The plan after the procedure was for Jin Jing to return to China, where she would update me on her progress with her doctors at home.

Four months after the treatment, Jing Jin wrote to me:

The miracle has appeared. I can walk slowly. I am very happy! The hand is also a bit more flexible than before, but it can't bend properly. I can't wash my hair myself, so I know that I should continue treatment. My forehead has recovered, it's completely fine, it's amazing.

I was thrilled with these initial results!

Then, six months after the first procedure, she wrote "the thing that makes me feel the most happy is that I can walk slowly with my child, as I hold her hand. Thank you for saving me and enabling me to stand up again."

In a second note she repeated, "Thank you again for saving me. This is something I never thought of: because I can stand up, I can take care of and accompany my child in the future, so that her childhood will not be missing. Thank you very much!"

Seeing the video of Jin Jing walking with her now five-year-old daughter and hearing stories like this are precisely what inspires me

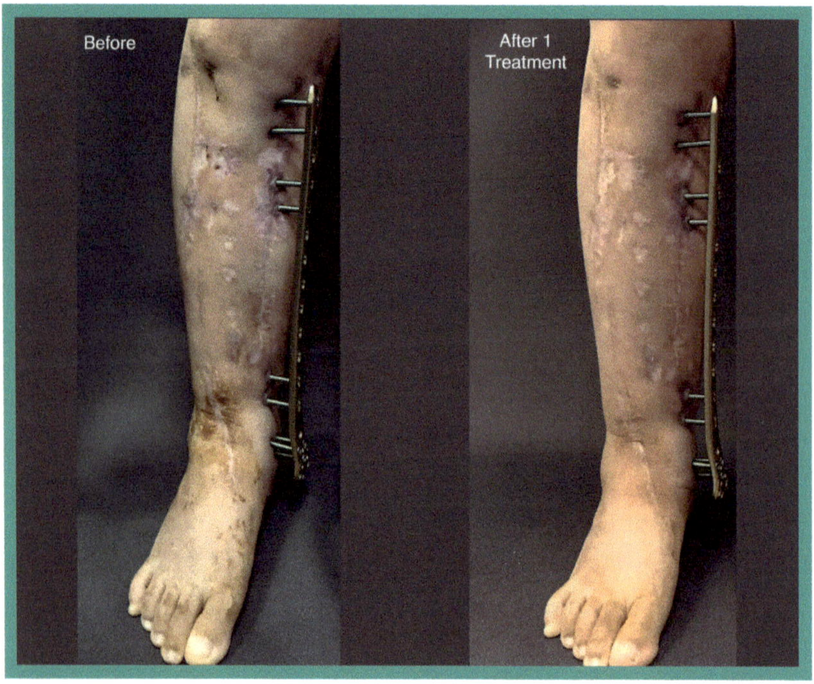

This is how Jin Jing arrived at our clinic, enduring the painful grip of an external fixator—a method to stabilize her shattered bones. Her doctors, seeing her leg not healing, recommended amputation. Even after one SCL treatment, you can see the visual skin and tissue improvements, but more importantly, Jin Jing is now able to walk with her daughter!

and drives my passion to continue my work on advancing stem cell therapy and technology.

When Jin Jing came back to see me seven months later for a second SCL procedure, I was elated to see that she no longer needed the wheelchair and could walk using a cane for support. Comparing her x-rays from before the initial procedure and six months after, it was clear that treatment was working. Her bones were healing, filling in the gap between the broken bones, thus enabling her to walk again.

Again using the SCL technique, I injected her own stem cells once more in the left upper leg, ankle, and foot, as well as in her forehead. I also took some hair from her scalp and used it for hair grafting to restore the missing eyebrow.

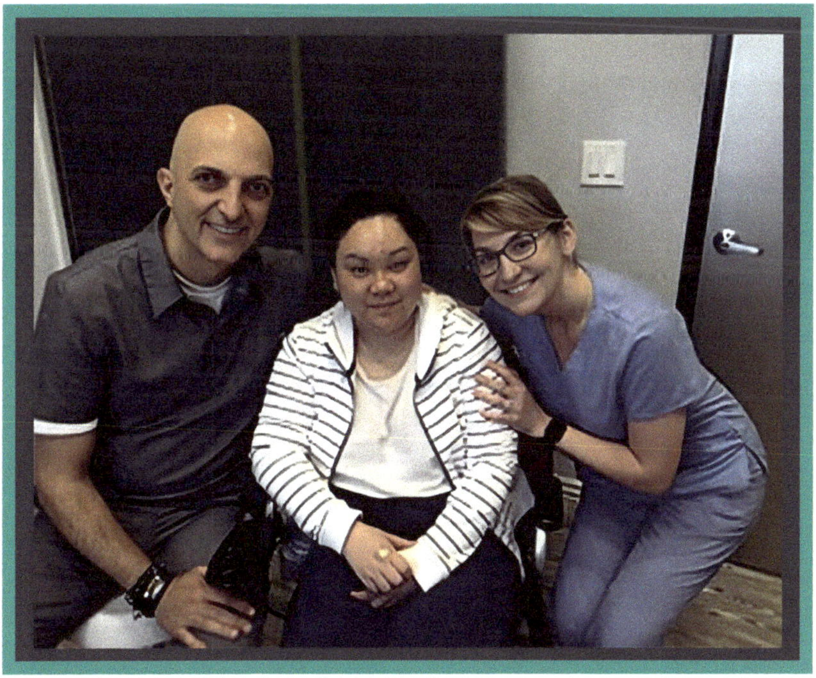

Jin Jing, arriving at my surgery center in Beverly Hills from China. During this time, her doctors recommended a leg amputation that would leave her wheelchair bound for the rest of her life. She found hope to save her from that.

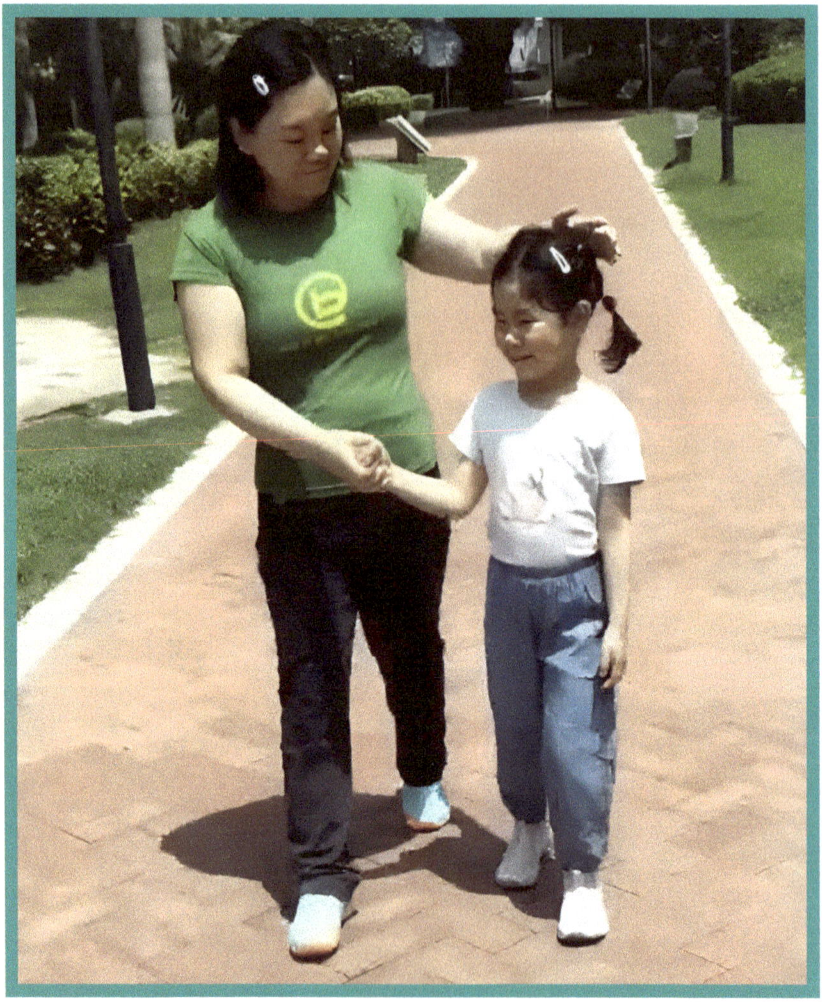

Two months after flying from China to Beverly Hills to receive my Stem Cell Lift, Jin Jing not only is able to walk without her wheelchair or crutches but can also walk with her beautiful daughter—a dream she thought would never come true before she we met.

After the procedure, she went to sleep at the hotel and the next day came to my medical center for post-op treatments to help optimize her healing and results and to reduce swelling and inflammation. She then returned home to China, promising to follow up with her doctors to take out the painful, uncomfortable, and unsightly metal screws that had been sticking out of her skin for the past three years.

Two months after her second SCL procedure, Jin Jing reported that she could now complete most of her daily activities, like washing her hair independently. Six months later, she had healed enough that the metal screws, which had become loose, could be removed from her leg. However, now it was in the middle of the COVID-19 pandemic, and she was told by her Chinese doctors that she should take out the loose screws by herself at home.

About a month later, the surgeons in China removed all the external fixation metals and remaining screws from her leg. A couple of months later, having recovered from this surgery, she sent me a video of her walking with her daughter in the park. A few months later, Jin Jing is living a full life, enjoying dancing, ice skating, and other activities.

Even now, Jin Jing's story is simply astonishing—and also a testament to the power of stem cells, when introduced optimally, to heal the body after even the most serious injury.

Reconstructive Healing

Stem cells have several mechanisms through which they can enhance reconstructive healing:

- **Cell replacement and regeneration.** Since stem cells have the ability to differentiate into specialized cell types that are needed for tissue repair, they are inherently suited to regeneration. Also, stem cells have a built-in homing mechanism that helps them to find the areas of injury and recognize the tissue in need of repair. The environment in which the stem cells find themselves dictates the response required. When transplanted into injured tissues like Jin Jing's legs and arms, stem cells signal the body to rebuild bone, literally replacing the damaged cells and restoring function.

- **Paracrine signaling.** Analogous to endocrine signaling via hormones, paracrine signaling via intercellular communication through the stroma found between cells is utilized to direct cellular function and balance. Stem cells do their job through a domino effect set off via the paracrine pathway by secreting chemical signals called secretomes that include growth factors, chemokines, cytokines, exosomes, liposomes, peptides, and other molecules that create a regenerative micro-environment that promotes healing and renewal. These secreted factors can stimulate nearby cells, including resident stem cells, to proliferate, differentiate, and migrate to the site of injury. Further, through the mechanism of paracrine signaling, stem cells are involved with modulating inflammation, enhancing angiogenesis (formation of new blood vessels), and promoting tissue remodeling and repair.
- **Extracellular matrix (ECM) modification.** Stem cells also help healing after injury by remodeling the ECM, which is the network of proteins (such as collagen) and molecules that provide structural support to tissues. Stem cells secrete enzymes and proteins that modify the composition and organization of the ECM, promoting cell migration, tissue integration, and the formation of functional tissue structures.
- **Angiogenesis and blood vessel formation.** Finally, stem cells have the ability to stimulate the growth of new blood vessels, which are crucial for supplying oxygen and nutrients to the injured areas.

Stem cells have enormous potential to be used in regenerative medicine as a reconstructive method in orthopedic, plastic, and neurosurgery. As you've seen throughout this chapter, stem cells have a powerful capacity to reconstruct bone, heal joint damage, and restore facial appearance after injury.

Stem cells have enormous potential to be used in regenerative medicine as a reconstructive method in orthopedic, plastic, and neurosurgery.

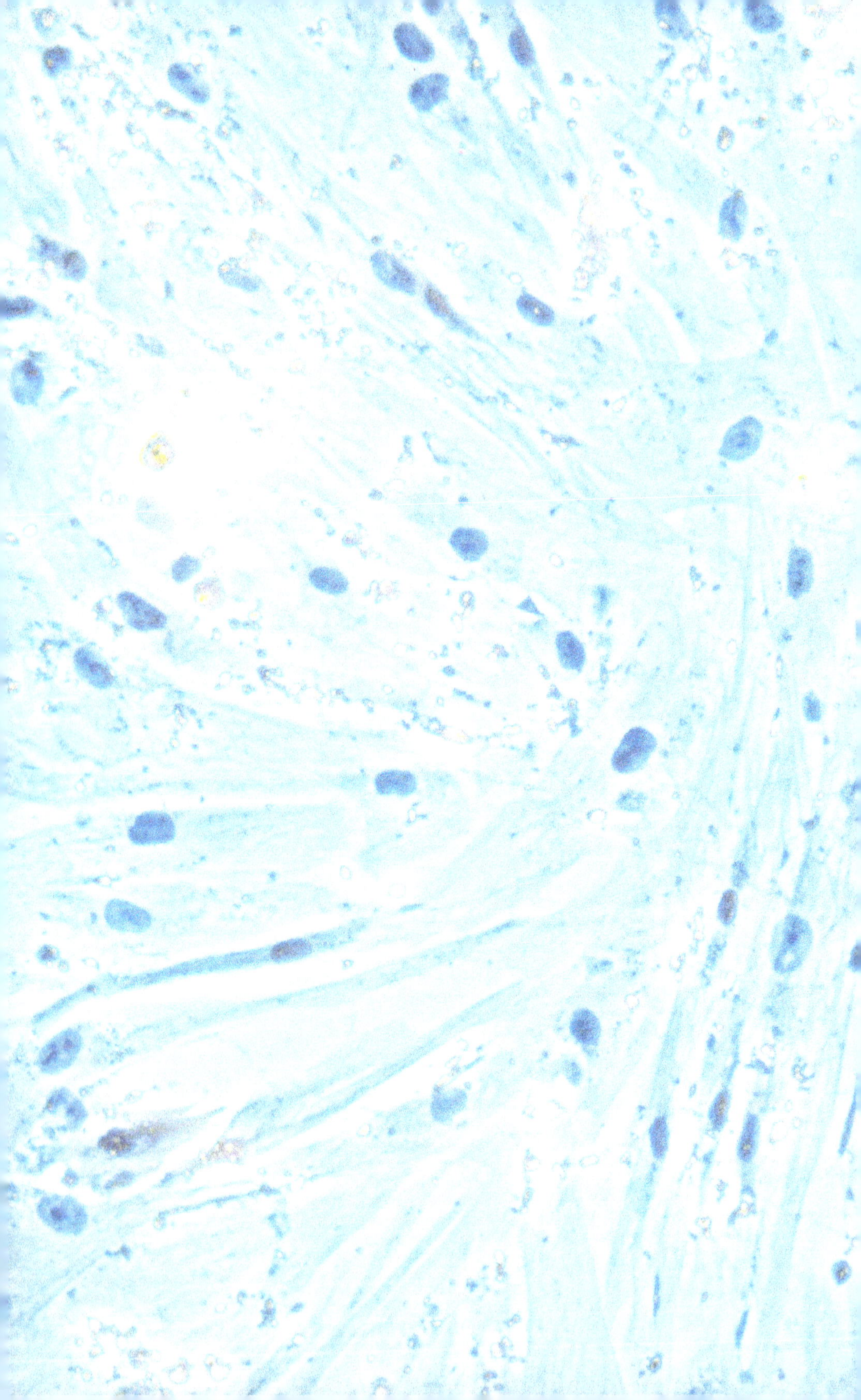

> *Searching and finding creative and innovative solutions for each patient intrigues me as a physician and gives me the utmost fulfillment.*

—DR. NATHAN NEWMAN

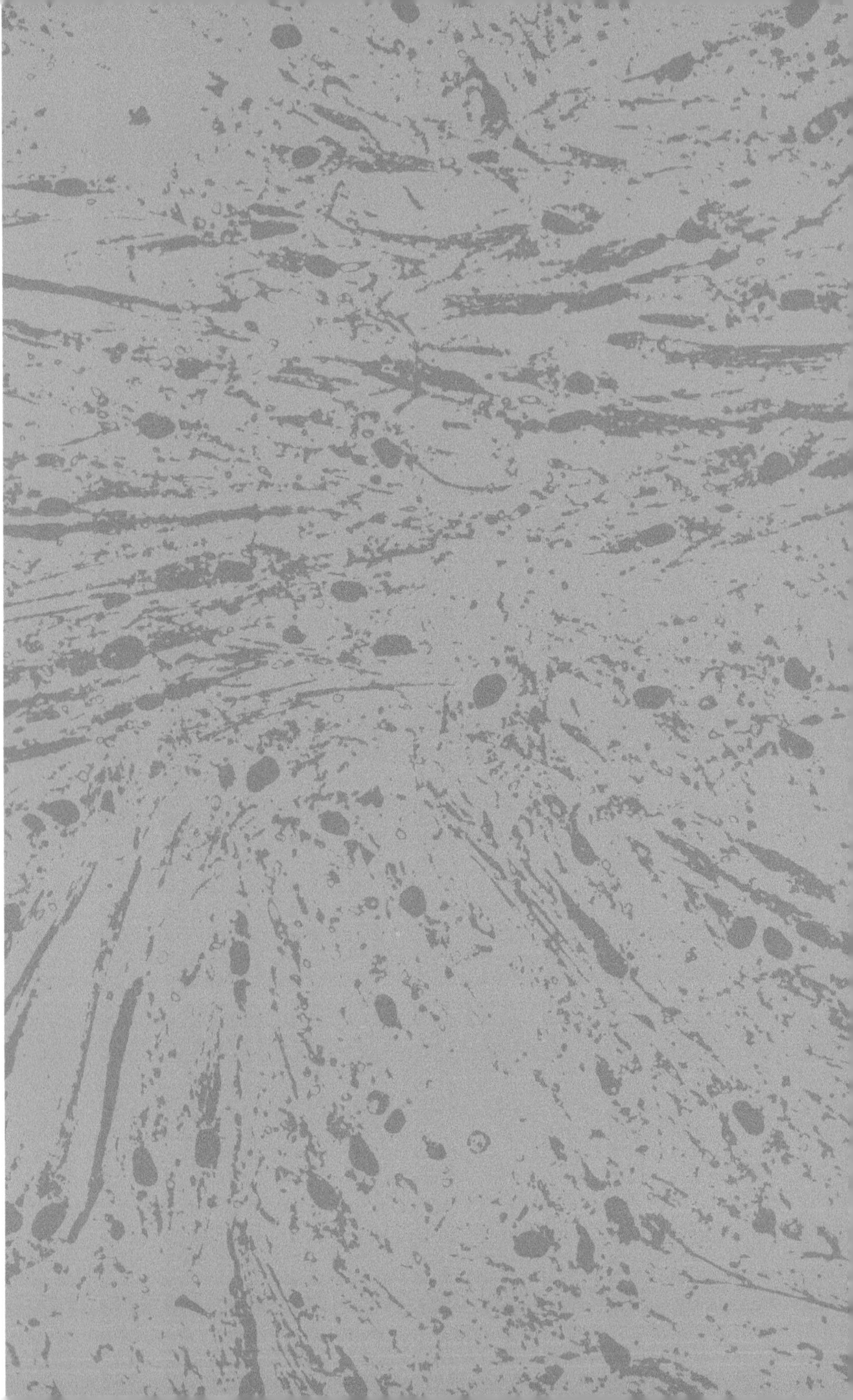

5

How the Stem Cell Lift Treats Lichen Sclerosus and Other Autoimmune Disorders

As the word spread about my work with stem cells, I received a phone call from a woman who had heard about my work with stem cells and had seen a video of the success I had treating Hersel. She said that she knew of a doctor in Italy who had used stem cells to treat lichen sclerosus. She asked hopelessly, "Have you heard of this disease?" Surprised to hear my positive reply that I am a dermatologist and, yes, I knew about her autoimmune skin condition, she quickly asked, "Do you think it can help? Can you treat me with stem cells?"

Meet Tammy: Stem Cells Work to Treat Lichen Sclerosus

Until this point, Tammy had been suffering in silence due to painful abrasions on her genitalia. For years, she had sought medical advice about the condition. Some doctors told her that it was "all in her head," while others diagnosed her with a candida rash and gave her antifungal medication. Still other physicians said she might have a sexually transmitted infection. None of these diagnoses was accurate. Tammy was suffering from an autoimmune condition called lichen sclerosus (LS).

"I'm in constant pain and can barely wear jeans, never mind a bathing suit. I've been to dozens of doctors and no one seems to understand what's going on or how to treat it. All I feel is ashamed and unheard—I feel hopeless."

I had never considered using my Stem Cell Lift procedure for this illness, but it made good sense. I then explained to Tammy that since stem cells have immunomodulatory capacity, they just might be able to get at one of the underlying factors of LS.

"You'd be my first lichen sclerosus patient," I said compassionately. "Are you willing to give it a go? I think my SCL procedure might provide you some relief and comfort."

Tammy responded with a resounding "Yes!" and we both smiled.

Once again, I was intrigued and wanted to do more research on this often-misdiagnosed condition and how stem cell therapy might be used for an autoimmune skin disease.

I knew that, as with most autoimmune disorders, the underlying or root cause of LS stemmed from a dysregulation of the immune system; something was not functioning as it should be. The immune system had mistaken this woman's cells as foreign and attacked the area. Whatever triggered the immune response had now set off a chronic assault on these tissues that waxed and waned but never fully let up, resulting in this debilitating condition.

Once I dove into the existing research, what really shocked me was the lack of medical data relating to LS. The medical books and scientific papers were not consistent or accurate about who can get the disease, what the symptoms are, and what worsens or improves the disease. As I read more, the treatment options were scanty at best; this information motivated me to devise a treatment that had the potential to give Tammy her life back.

I knew that stem cells throughout the body were in constant communication with the immune system, so my question became, could I use stem cells to calm down Tammy's immune system so it wouldn't cause the flare-ups? Would it be possible to control the autoimmune process while healing her damaged tissues?

The Stem Cell Lift treatment had given my patient back her autonomy and released her from a life of pain and shame.

And that's exactly what happened. Using my SCL procedure, harvesting Tammy's own stem cells from her fat tissue, concentrating them, and reintroducing them very gently and carefully into her genital area gave her immediate relief. After years of suffering, her pain subsided, the swelling and irritation decreased, and, within days, she was able to wear jeans and cross her legs again. Within a few weeks, she was able to resume intimacy with her husband without her genital skin tearing. Her treatment had improved the atrophied tissue, released fused tissues, and restored a healthy tissue color. In essence, the SCL treatment had given her back her autonomy and released her from a life of pain and shame.

Given Tammy's success, I was spurred on to learn more about LS and continue to refine my SCL technique for LS to personalize and optimize results for individual patients.

More LS Patients Find Me

Soon after I successfully treated Tammy, a number of other women suffering from LS would soon become my patients as the word spread through online LS support groups. Thousands of women were finding one another and connecting online to share their frustrations and exchange stories, experiences, and recommendations about the pain and discomfort caused by this often-misdiagnosed condition.

Another woman reached out to me to learn about the SCL for LS. Karen was a woman in her mid-30s, a wife, and a mother of two children. As she described, "I have an adoring husband and I've been looking at an existence without a sex life. My constant vaginal pain has been so intense that even sitting down or walking can make me cry. The pain is so throbbing that even standing beyond 30 minutes at a time is simply excruciating."

Then Karen described what another doctor had diagnosed her with.

"The doctor told me that I probably had gonorrhea or chlamydia. I was in shock. I was embarrassed, ashamed, and concerned at the same time. I was a faithful wife; I didn't cheat. Never. That only meant one thing—my supposed 'devoted' husband had cheated on me!"

As Karen recounted this scene from her previous doctor's visit, I could see all the guilt, confusion, and fear pass across her face as she wiped away tears.

When Karen shared this with me, I felt immediately concerned and wanted to help her out of her misery.

Karen continued, "I confronted my husband who told me that no way did he have an STD like that. He reassured me that he had been faithful to me. His words took a moment to sink in. For a few minutes, I held onto a small negative doubt in my mind, but after a minute or two of playback in my memory, I knew it was the truth. We've never had any major issues. My 'spider sense' never tingled over his behavior. No, neither of us had been unfaithful."

After examining her to confirm a diagnosis of lichen sclerosus and to understand the extent of her condition, we talked about the SCL procedure. Since Karen's condition was so severe, I had to lower her expectations about how effective the procedure would be in her case.

I explained that she may require multiple treatments spaced three to six months apart. She should see improvement in her symptoms with each treatment, and her recovery should be easier as the health of the tissues improves. The aim was to reduce or eliminate the debilitating symptoms and discomfort that was limiting and impeding her from doing what most of us take for granted in our daily lives.

Thankfully, once again, the results for Karen were almost immediate: about a week after the procedure, she was able to dress and move about without pain. With three treatments, she achieved clinical remission of her LS and became symptom-free.

"I can't believe it," she said, in tears of joy this time. "Putting on my pants didn't hurt. I feel like this whole experience is like something out of an 'old-time' Hollywood movie. It's like a miracle! The pain is gone and it all happened in a flash!"

I was beyond thrilled with Karen's response. At her next appointment, Karen admitted, "It didn't seem real at first. It only felt surreal. The years of pain, discomfort, and emotional turmoil had been dissolved away in a moment."

Tears welled up in her eyes, and even Nualla, my compassionate nurse, looked concerned.

"What's wrong, Karen?" asked my nurse. "Are you okay?"

"Yes," Karen replied. "I don't know what to say . . . the pain is just gone."

Urged by Tammy, Karen, and other patients, we set up a LS Facebook group for our patients. I was very interested in understanding more about this disease and also in collecting data resulting from my treatment approach, specifically with the outcomes of my SCL procedure. Along with my research team, I led and carried out a retrospective clinical study of 111 women ages 20 to 76 who had undergone the SCL procedure at our clinic from 2011 to 2015.

My study, which was a follow up to a 2015 article I had published in the *Medical Journal of Obstetrics and Gynecology*, proved that I was on the right track: the results achieved with three treatments of stem cells derived from patients' own fat tissue and reintroduced had dramatically improved patient LS symptoms and quality of life, and even restored structural anatomy in some. Patients were able to engage in intercourse and comfortably wear underwear and tight-fitting pants like jeans, and reported an overall decrease of symptoms. It was clear: stem cell therapy was a powerful immune modulator. My study also revealed that early intervention may help prevent damage and/or restore normal anatomy. The results of this study were published in a 2018 paper, entitled "Autologous Adipose-Derived Stem Cell Treatment for Women with Genital Lichen Sclerosus."[1]

The results achieved with three treatments of stem cells derived from patients' own fat tissue and reintroduced had dramatically improved patient LS symptoms and quality of life, and even restored structural anatomy in some.

As additional LS patients sought out my treatment, I continued to improve my treatment protocols based on their experience and data. My medical team and I continue to follow our patients to this day. Indeed, I have changed the goal of the stem cell lift treatments from merely providing some comfort and improvement to my LS patients to our goal today of achieving remission of disease in these patients. I continue to research and publish my findings in order to bring awareness and solutions for the treatment of LS. And now, almost 15 years after I first treated Tammy, I have helped hundreds of women suffering from LS achieve remission from their autoimmune disease.

Understanding Lichen Sclerosus

Lichen sclerosus et atrophicus, now just called lichen sclerosus, is a chronic inflammatory autoimmune disorder of the skin usually involving the genital and anal areas. As with many autoimmune disorders, LS is actually a spectrum of disease, and its symptoms include dyspareunia (painful intercourse) and pelvic floor dysfunction. The disease is most prevalent in women, followed by men, and rarely, children. Although there is no one determined cause for this devastating disease, it is hypothesized that patients possessing a genetic predisposition to developing a "misdirected" immune response may develop a localized autoimmune response from certain triggers, such as infection, stress, hormonal changes, or trauma. Because of old and outdated misconceptions that are still in medical textbooks and literature, there is continued confusion around the disease and an often-extended delay in correctly diagnosing the condition.

It is not clear how many people are afflicted with this condition; the estimated prevalence of the disease is as high as 1 in 300 patients. (Diabetes in 2024 is about 1 out of 20.) Most cases of LS are diagnosed by dermatologists and gynecologists. The symptoms vary dramatically. Patients may have no physical symptoms, but their physical examination may reveal active and advanced disease, or vice versa—the physical examination appears almost normal, but the patient is experiencing excruciating pain, constant burning, itching, and tearing that cannot be relieved with prescribed medications. Some patients describe it as feeling like bees are constantly stinging them or ants are crawling under their skin. The tears on genitalia range from small papercuts to deep fissures, erosions, and blisters. Many women experience loss of normal anatomy, fusing of the labia minora, phimosis (where the clitoris is buried under the clitoral hood, causing reduced sensation), narrowing of the vaginal opening, and scarring of the tissues, as well as a thinning of the skin so severe that a wipe of toilet paper will cause painful rupture or tearing of the skin. Although LS may cause significant pain and discomfort, it doesn't affect the inner reproductive organs, such as the vaginal canal or the uterus.

Because of these symptoms, patients have to severely curtail their lifestyle: they cannot wear underwear or jeans; they cannot stand or sit for extended periods of time; they cannot exercise or have sexual intercourse. Dealing with such severe symptoms often triggers mental health issues, including anxiety and depression, with some women contemplating suicide. And yet, despite the extremity of these symptoms, many women go undiagnosed or misdiagnosed for years, exacerbating their physical condition and the toll it has on their personal lives and that of their loved ones.

In men, the term *balanitis xerotica obliterans* (BXO) is used to describe lichen sclerosus of the penis. Men who develop LS are usually uncircumcised, and the foreskin can become tight, shrunken, and scarred over the head of the penis. LS in men may result in difficulty pulling back the foreskin, decreased sensation at the tip of the penis, painful erections, or problems with urination.

Less commonly, extragenital LS (lesions on the skin outside the genitalia) appears on the back, chest, breasts, or arms and is not symptomatic. Extragenital LS appears to be more common in women and may affect one in five LS patients. These lesions tend to be white, flat or raised, and not as itchy as the affected skin of the genitals or anus.

While there are thousands of LS sufferers, many doctors are not familiar enough with the disease, and therefore, are not able to diagnose it correctly. Many patients self-diagnose through online research or are forced to see numerous doctors before a correct diagnosis is made. For LS, as with many other chronic skin diseases, there are limited effective medical treatments to manage the disease. In most cases, doctors prescribe a strong corticosteroid ointment or cream to provide temporary relief of the itching and discomfort.

Incidence of Lichen Sclerosus Compared to Other Diseases

In the general population, the cumulative incidence of LS over a 20-year period is approximately 1.54 percent (15.4 per 1,000 people). For females, it's 2.13 percent, and for males, it's 0.97 percent.[2] Incredibly, it's characterized as rare, but it has an astonishingly high rate of incidence compared to most common diseases:

Rheumatoid arthritis (RA) In 2021, the global age-standardized incidence rate (ASIR) of RA among AYAs was 9.46 per 100,000 population. The age-standardized prevalence rate (ASPR) was 104.35 per 100,000 population. The age-standardized mortality rate (ASMR) was 0.016 per 100,000 population.[3]

Inflammatory bowel disease (IBD) The ASIR for IBD in AYAs was 4.08, with an ASPR of 29.55 and an ASMR of 0.10.[4]

Multiple sclerosis (MS) MS exhibited an ASIR of 1.40, an ASPR of 16.05, and an ASMR of 0.05.

Type 1 diabetes mellitus (T1DM) T1DM had an ASIR of 6.63, an ASPR of 245.51, and an ASMR of 0.54.[5]

Asthma Asthma showed an ASIR of 232.22, an ASPR of 2245.51, and an ASMR of 0.89.[6]

Psoriasis Psoriasis had an ASIR of 55.08 and an ASPR of 426.16.

As with other autoimmune diseases, LS patients are also more prone to developing other autoimmune disorders such as thyroid disease, gastrointestinal disease, lichen planus, vitiligo, and interstitial cystitis. Many patients also have hormonal imbalances that drive the dysregulation of the immune system and exacerbate their condition.

The Symptoms of Lichen Sclerosus in Women

Although some patients experience symptoms only of the vulvar area, most patients suffer from symptoms in the vulvar and perianal area, including the following:

- Vulvar itching (this is the most common symptom and may be so severe that it interferes with sleep or wearing pants)
- Fissures
- Bleeding
- Pain
- Burning sensation
- Discomfort or pain (vulvodynia)
- Soreness
- Tearing
- Blisters
- Painful sexual intercourse (dyspareunia) as a result of repeated cracking or tearing of the skin (fissuring) or from narrowing of the vaginal opening due to scarring

Unfortunately, women with LS are often misdiagnosed, and it can be years before they get some relief from the pain and discomfort, both physical and emotional. Since many doctors are not familiar with LS, they often mistake the symptoms for yeast infections, a herpes outbreak, low estrogen and normal post-menopausal changes, vitiligo, or, even more devastating, evidence of a psychological disorder. LS is not contagious.

Making matters worse, the diagnosis of LS may not be made until the disease has advanced and altered the normal anatomy of the genitalia. Early in the disease, small, white, shiny and smooth spots appear on the skin and mucosa in the genital and anal areas. Many patients do not initially notice the disease, as they may not have any symptoms. As the disease progresses, the spots grow into bigger patches and the skin becomes thin and crinkled. Patients complain of disconcerting changes to their skin, including bright red or purple bruises and white or dark patches. These topical changes reflect the skin becoming fragile, tearing easily with the slightest friction.

Many of my patients suffered for years before discovering both an accurate diagnosis and hope for relief with the SCL procedure.

Without effective treatment, these changes cause a state of chronic inflammation that can result in scarring of the tissues and ultimately structural changes to anatomy. Fusing of the labia minora to the labia majora, narrowing of the vaginal opening, and scarring over the clitoris are common signs of the disease's progression.

Many of my patients suffered for years before discovering both an accurate diagnosis and hope for relief with the SCL procedure.

The Limitations of Common Treatments for LS

The severity of LS varies from person to person. Most individuals experience flare-ups, which may be associated with hormonal changes, trauma, or periods of physical or emotional stress. During a flare-up, the LS symptoms become more severe, and tissue damage, alterations, or scarring may be rapid. Typically, these outbreaks have been treated with potent topical corticosteroids in hopes of reducing inflammation, providing symptomatic comfort, and minimizing tissue damage.

This treatment usually provides some symptomatic relief but does not address the source of the problem. In fact, many women experience minimal relief or even more irritation with long-term steroid treatment.

In order to treat LS more comprehensively, it's important to find a physician who can diagnose it correctly. In most cases, an experienced physician can make a diagnosis based on the history of the course of the disease and the clinical appearance of affected areas. Some doctors may want to conduct a biopsy to confirm the diagnosis. It is important to note that if the biopsy doesn't confirm the disease, it doesn't necessarily mean that the patient doesn't have LS; it may simply be that the spot that was biopsied does not show the classical changes of the disease. The physician may also conduct tests to confirm or exclude other conditions that could cause symptoms similar to those of LS, such as:

- Lichen planus, a skin disease that can also cause itching and fusing of the genital skin and can occur together with LS
- Low estrogen level, which can cause vaginal dryness, thinning of tissues, and painful intercourse
- Vitiligo, an autoimmune skin disorder that can cause white skin patches similar to those of LS and that can occur together with LS

- Pemphigoid, a rare blistering skin disorder that also causes scarring of the vulva
- Hemorrhoids, which can also cause cracks in the skin of the anus

Men who have LS are generally treated with circumcision, as removing the foreskin of the penis has shown to significantly resolve LS symptoms. Until now, the standard of care for treating LS has been the use of potent corticosteroids such as clobetasol. The anti-inflammatory effect of the medication may help alleviate symptoms and reduce the damage to the tissues in the short term. However, chronic long-term use of this medication may result in thinning of the tissues, exacerbating the symptoms of the disease and creating a precarious dependence on the drug such that when it is discontinued abruptly, a rebound flare can result. This becomes a vicious cycle of steroid dependence, as "the flare" from steroid "withdrawal" is difficult to differentiate from that of LS. When this happens, the tissues need to be weaned off the steroids gradually to prevent the rebound flare reaction. Laser, radiofrequency, and focused ultrasound treatments also have been used to address the symptoms of LS but with little long-term success, as these treatments may result in reduced blood flow and cause scarring of the tissues. Ultimately, these treatments do not address the disease but merely try to reduce the symptoms temporarily.

Other treatments that have been less commonly used but have shown benefits for some patients include hormonal replacement therapy (HRT), prescriptive immune modulators such as tacrolimus, low-dose naltrexone, and light or non-ablative laser treatments. These may provide some relief from the symptoms of LS but usually do not stop the progression of the disease. Finally, surgical vaginal reconstruction has been used to cut and remove scar tissue and to improve the structural appearance of the female genitalia; however, there are many risks and complications associated with this procedure. More importantly, the symptoms of LS may even get worse after surgical repair.

All that said, up until the SCL procedure, there had been no effective treatment for LS.

Treating LS with the Stem Cell Lift

The SCL method delivers an enhanced amount of stem cells found in the patient's own fat to the affected areas. These cells are tasked with reducing inflammation, improving circulation, repairing the collagen scaffolding, restoring elasticity, and repairing damaged cells and tissues. In many cases, I have seen almost immediate changes and improvement in symptoms from the effects of the stem cell secretory factors that are released into the tissues. The SCL treatment is the only method that has been documented to achieve complete relief of symptoms and stop the progression of LS.

The SCL treatment is the only method that has been documented to achieve complete relief of symptoms and stop the progression of LS.

I consider patients who, in effect, become "disease-free" to have achieved autoimmune remission, much like with cancer treatment. The autoimmune response may be mitigated through the effects of the stem cells, which may take about three months after the procedure to attach and become permanently incorporated into their new surroundings. They may continue to improve the tissues for about one year after the procedure. To date, about one in three patients has achieved remission with the SCL procedure. This means they are symptom-free and do not need to use medications on a regular basis; their anatomy is stable and no longer shows disease activity.

The remaining two-thirds of the patients report marked improvement in their symptoms, with noted reduction in pain, burning, and itching and improved look and feel of the anatomy of the treated areas. Patients treated with the SCL procedure report having less frequent, shorter flare-ups with far less intense pain and discomfort. Most patients are able to discontinue the use of topical steroids and are able to resume intimacy and sexual intercourse. Patients experience improvement with each treatment but may need to have a series of treatments (usually two or three) to achieve the desired improvement and relief from LS symptoms.

I have also found a correlation between LS and low estrogen and other hormonal imbalances in many of my patients, which can influence their immune response and health. So, I often consider including hormone balancing therapy with bioidentical hormones as part of my treatment protocol.

The SCL works because it:

- Uses stem cells, which can turn off autoimmune dysregulation and put the disease into remission
- Uses your own body's cells that are genetically tasked with repair, restoration, and maintenance of tissues
- Reduces pain and discomfort from scar contraction through scar remodeling
- Improves and relieves signs and symptoms of LS
- Provides immune modulating activity that may diminish or stop the autoimmune reaction
- May be repeated as needed and has additive effects with each treatment

- May be combined with platelet-rich plasma (PRP)
- May alleviate the need for topical treatments (e.g., steroids and immune modulators like tacrolimus)

And it is:

- Natural
- Not a drug
- Not a hormone
- Autologous, from your own body
- Not rejected by the body

And it requires:

- No allergy testing
- No incisions (cuts)
- No sutures
- No general anesthesia
- Minimal downtime or recovery period

How Stem Cell Therapy Can Help Other Autoimmune Disorders

Researchers are looking at how stem cell therapy can successfully address other autoimmune conditions. Autoimmune diseases occur when the immune system attacks normal tissues of the body. The immune system normally provides protection against germs, such as bacteria and viruses, and immediately activates the defense cells upon detecting these. In an autoimmune disease, the immune system perceives the body's various tissues and organs, such as joints and skin, as foreign. For example, type 1 diabetes, which is an autoimmune disease, attacks pancreatic cells, and rheumatoid arthritis attacks joints. A healthy immune system knows the difference between foreign invaders and the body's own cells, organs, and "good" microorganisms.

Autoimmune diseases are mostly provoked by the tissues presenting something as foreign to the immune system. Unfortunately, there are over 100 different types of autoimmune diseases, but some of them occur more frequently, including rheumatoid arthritis (RA), multiple sclerosis (MS), juvenile idiopathic arthritis (JIA), systemic sclerosis (SS), diabetes mellitus type 1, systemic lupus erythematosus (SLE), inflammatory bowel disease, and Addison's disease.

> It is my great hope that other doctors and scientists will look at the enormous potential of stem cell therapy to address autoimmune disorders. Indeed, recently, stem cells have been found to be effective in treating a range of autoimmune illnesses in both in vitro and in vivo investigations. LS is just the beginning!

It is my great hope that other doctors and scientists will look at the enormous potential of stem cell therapy to address autoimmune disorders. Indeed, recently, stem cells have been found to be effective in treating a range of autoimmune illnesses in both in vitro and in vivo investigations. LS is just the beginning!

> *“Stem cells hold the potential to become specialized cells and integrate and repair any tissue in the body.”*
>
> –DR. NATHAN NEWMAN

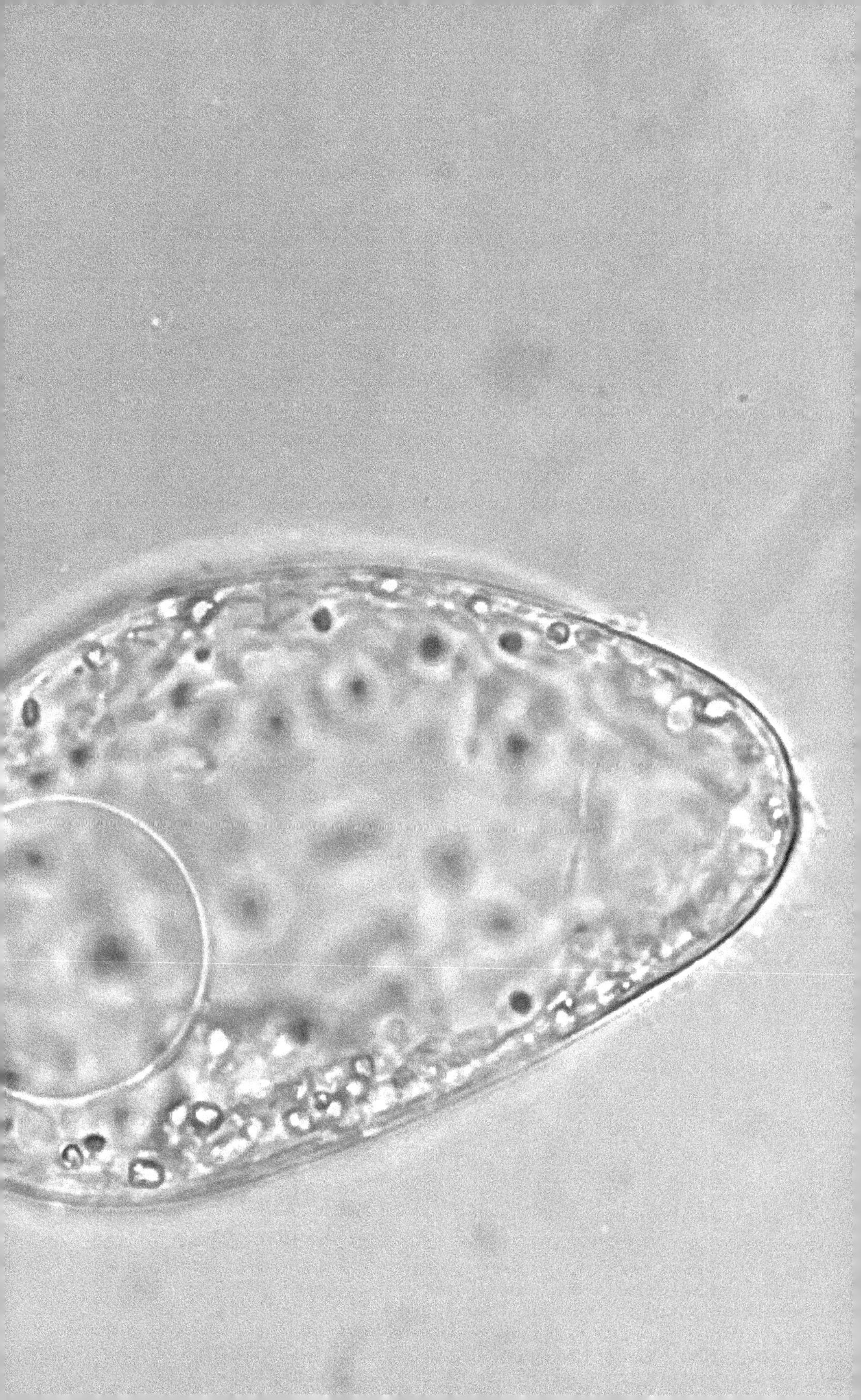

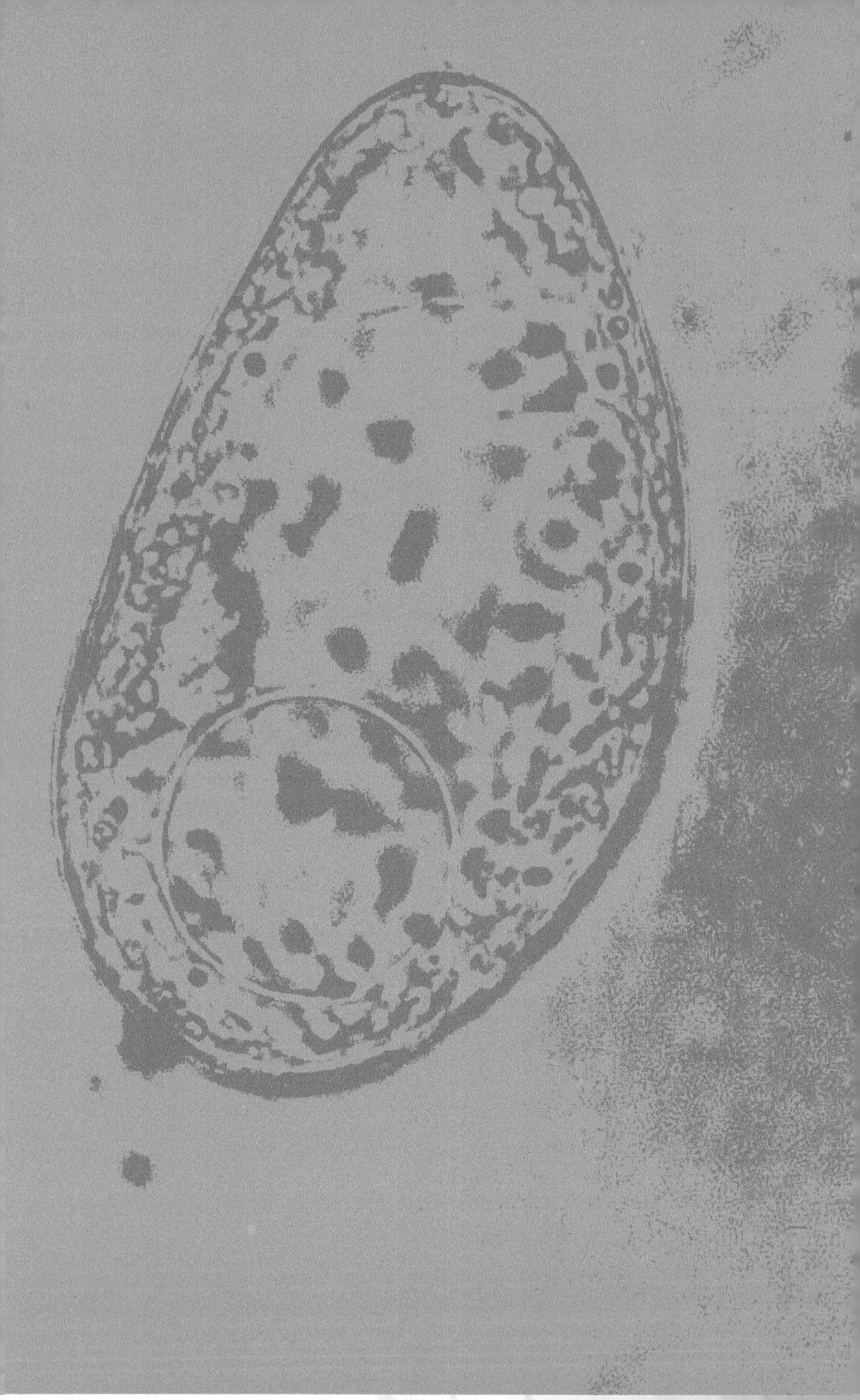

6

How the Stem Cell Lift Improves Musculoskeletal Conditions

As you've seen with patients needing tissue repair and reconstruction, as well as those suffering from debilitating autoimmune skin diseases like lichen sclerosus, the Stem Cell Lift procedure is enormously versatile, offering people many ways to reclaim fulfilling lives.

Meet Chuck: Professional Prize Fighter

Chuck Liddell, a world-renowned mixed martial arts prize fighter (he was a UFC light heavyweight champion) sought me out, hoping that I might help him. After years of wear and tear, Chuck's knees were in bad shape. He was also in constant pain. Like many professional elite-level athletes, Chuck was suffering from chronic joint pain in his left knee.

When he came into my office for his first exam, he explained that he had to "fight to stabilize" his leg. His MRI showed that the meniscus (the C-shaped cartilage padding between the bones) on the side of his left knee was torn. The MRI also showed that he had strains and tears in the ligaments in and around his knee. No wonder he was in so much pain!

After I described the SCL procedure, and he was game to give it a try. I explained how I would first extract fat cells from his body, separate the stem cells from the fat cells, concentrate the stem cells, and then reintroduce them into his knee and the areas around it. I predicted that the stem cells would help take down the inflammation and heal the tear in the meniscus and the tendons—which would not only

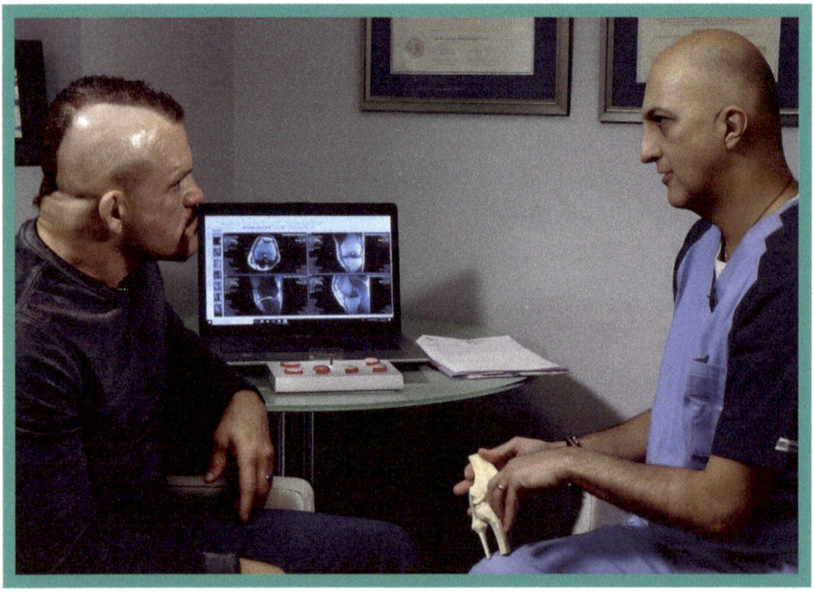

UFC champion Chuck Liddell couldn't afford the downtime and risks of traditional surgery, so he opted for my innovative Stem Cell Lift to alleviate the pain of injuries sustained throughout his career.

lessen the pain and discomfort but also allow the tendon and the cartilage to heal naturally.

Typically, athletes with sports injuries undergo an invasive orthopedic surgery to treat such ligament tears and joint issues; such surgical procedures not only are invasive—often involving trimming the damaged part of the meniscus, for instance—but also require a long time to heal before the patient is able to get back to normal activities.

Right after the procedure, Chuck exclaimed, "I already feel the difference!"

And two months later, he was back training.

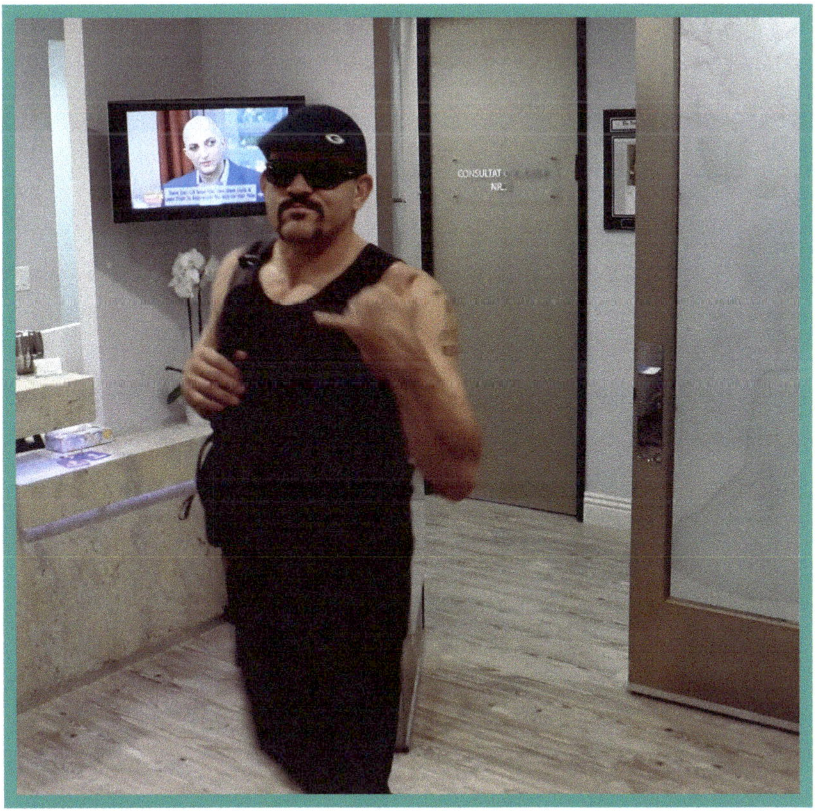

Three months after Chuck's SCL, he is back to training as he did years ago. He says, "It works. I don't know what else to say, it just works. It's done a great deal of good for me."

I asked Chuck to come and see me after three months so that I could evaluate whether or not he might benefit from a second round of treatments. When he came to see me, however, he told me he was doing awesome.

"I can even sit back on my knees! I haven't been able to do that in years!"

Clearly, the SCL had worked wonders for Chuck.

Meet Bas: World-Famous Martial Artist and Actor

Bas Rutten, the world-famous mixed martial artist and actor from Holland, had had an extensive career as a fighter. A former UFC

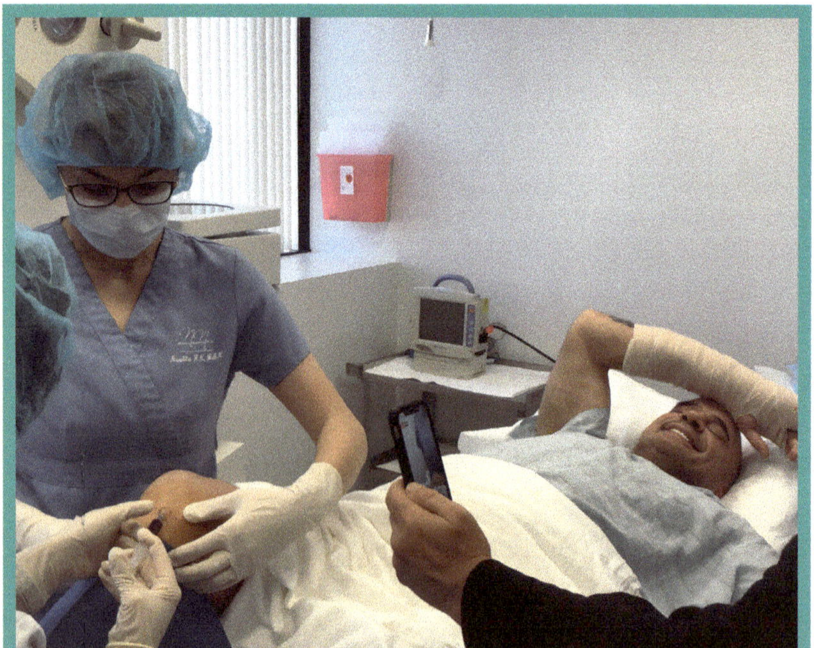

Legendary UFC champion Bas Rutten, with 34 professional fights under his belt, endured significant damage to his knees. Unwilling to face the risks of a knee replacement, he chose a Stem Cell Lift.

heavyweight champion and Hall of Famer, he had achieved legendary status in the sport. Now, after years of grappling with the lasting effects of multiple injuries, he wanted to see if the SCL could help him achieve more holistic healing so that he was not in such constant pain. In our first meeting, Bas told me proudly that he'd been in 34 professional fights. It was no surprise that he'd suffered a lot of injuries over the years and that his joints had also taken a beating.

When he came to see me, I asked him about his concerns, physical problems, and limitations he had with his knees; took a look at the MRI of both knees; and examined him. As with many lean athletes, Bas did not have any areas from which I could get fat. I explained that since he did not have much body fat, I would take the stem cells from his bone marrow instead, and I felt confident that the stem cell procedure would benefit him. I described the needle aspiration of the stem cells found in the bone marrow of his hip bone.

He agreed, and I injected Bas's own stem cells into his knee joint and the tissue around his knee to repair the damaged joints and ligaments and help alleviate the pain from the chronic inflammation and worn-down cartilage.

Immediately after the procedure, Bas got up and said, "I can walk!" He couldn't believe that he could just walk off the procedure table and change back into his clothes without experiencing pain. He also had no need to be immobilized or go through the pain and lengthy recovery of surgery. He was experiencing a new kind of treatment like he had never experienced before.

Throughout my 25 years of practice, I've treated thousands of people from all walks of life. From ordinary people to professional athletes, from young teenagers to elderly patients, the vast majority of them felt better after the SCL as their symptoms got milder or resolved completely. Some wanted to buy time before undergoing a major surgery such as a knee replacement, and some were seeking an alternative solution to resolve their medical problem altogether.

As with most of the SCL procedures, the stem cell procedure took about three months to have their permanent effect; this three-month window reflects the time it takes for the stem cells to graft to the tissue and create permanent results, building back tissue where it was lost or injured. Even after this initial healing period, the stem cells will continue to improve, repair, and regenerate tissues for about a year after the procedure.

The SCL procedure enables the body to begin its own natural healing process; reduces the time it takes for the body to heal; and avoids the need for surgery and joint replacement as well as drugs and pain

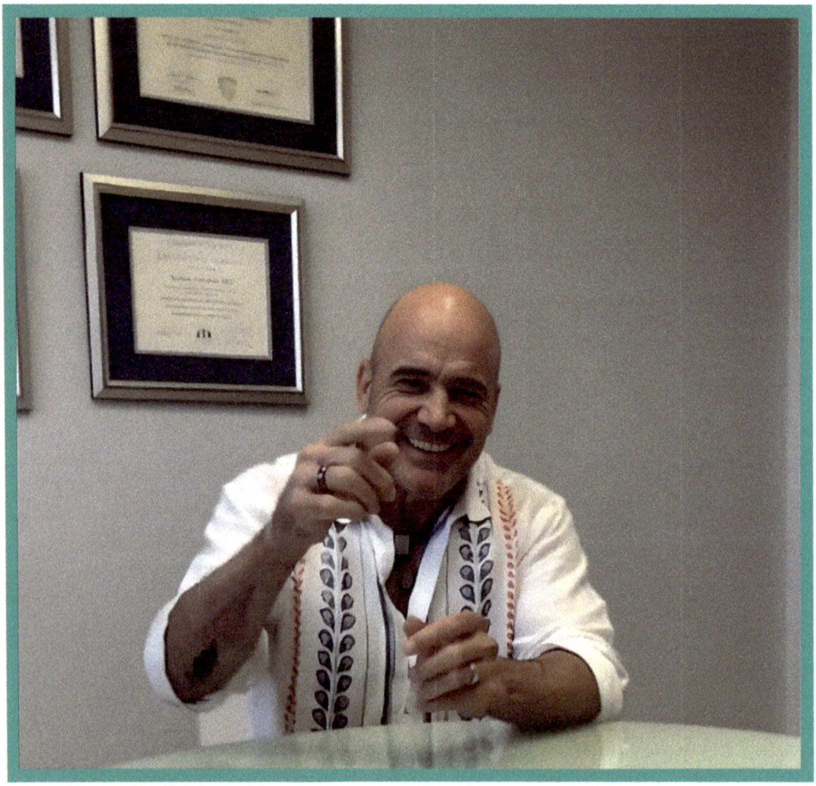

Three months after the SCL, Bas is absolutely thrilled with his results, proclaiming, "Now I can walk again. The results are really phenomenal."

relievers, which may hurt the liver or kidneys and cause the stomach to bleed. The SCL causes none of these side effects; it is safe and effective, offering people lasting results.

> The SCL procedure enables the body to begin its own natural healing process; reduces the time it takes for the body to heal; and avoids the need for surgery and joint replacement as well as drugs and pain relievers, which may hurt the liver or kidneys and cause the stomach to bleed.

Stem Cell Therapy for Arthritis

Many athletes suffer from similar joint problems. Typically, sports injuries affect the knees, ankles, shoulders, and hands. And if they don't have acute injuries, many athletes develop arthritis after years of wear and tear. Indeed, osteoarthritis (OA) is the most common chronic condition of the joints, affecting more than 30 million adults in the United States alone. OA is a degenerative disease of the joints that occurs when the cartilage or cushion between the joints breaks down, leading to pain, swelling, and stiffness. Some risk factors include joint injury or overuse, gender, obesity, race, genetics, and age—it is highly prevalent among the elderly. Symptoms include pain, swelling, and stiffness.

In addition to treating OA, the SCL can also be used to heal the symptoms of another type of arthritis—rheumatoid arthritis (RA). Unlike osteoarthritis, RA is an autoimmune condition in which the immune system attacks the joints and creates inflammation that causes the tissues that line the joint to thicken. This results in swelling and pain in and around the joints, leading to joint destruction, disfigurement, and permanent disability. I've treated numerous patients suffering from RA in their hands. In fact, one woman came in for the SCL cosmetic procedure to address wrinkles and sagging skin on her face, neck, and hands. She also happened to suffer from painful RA in her hands, which limited her ability to carry out normal daily tasks. With the SCL procedure, I was able to simultaneously address both her cosmetic and medical concerns, rejuvenating her appearance and alleviating her RA symptoms. She was very pleased to be pain-free and to see improvement in the two areas that are most revealing clues to one's age: the face and hands.

> Regardless of whether the arthritis is OA or RA, stem cell injections through the SCL method can alleviate the symptoms related to inflammation, including swelling, pain, and lack of mobility.

Regardless of whether the arthritis is OA or RA, stem cell injections through the SCL method can alleviate the symptoms related to inflammation, including swelling, pain, and lack of mobility.

Understanding Inflammatory Arthritis

Inflammatory arthritis refers to a group of conditions affecting joints that are all rooted in a dysregulation of the immune system. When joints are inflamed, patients experience pain, stiffness, and lack of mobility. Joints can also swell and feel tender to the touch, which again will restrict movement. It's important to note that though inflammatory arthritis primarily affects the joints, it can also affect other tissues in the body, including the heart, lungs, skin, and other organs. These ancillary or downstream effects point to the importance of early treatment.

While it's not known what causes inflammatory arthritis in every patient, what is known is that it's rooted in the immune system mistakenly attacking normal tissues. Normally, when we are exposed to pathogens such as bacteria, viruses, or fungi, the immune system produces white blood cells called lymphocytes as well as immune proteins to mount an attack against these invaders. Lymphocytes and immune proteins then signal the tissues to trigger inflammation, which helps defend against infection; this is a short-term response that resolves quickly.

However, when a patient's immune system does not function properly, they may suffer from chronic inflammation, a condition in which the immune response does not know how or when to stop the assault, resulting in long-term damage to the tissues. Malfunction in the immune response system begins to attack a patient's own tissues instead of the foreign invader, which is why we call it an autoimmune response.

As we saw in the previous chapter on lichen sclerosus, stem cells help to harmonize (or modulate) a malfunctioning immune response, which is so important to treating and controlling autoimmune conditions.

The Prevalence of Musculoskeletal Conditions

According to the World Health Organization (WHO), approximately 1.71 billion people worldwide suffer from one of several musculoskeletal conditions. Stem cell therapy, especially the SCL procedure, offers physicians and patients noninvasive, safe treatment options. As the WHO points out:[1]

- Musculoskeletal conditions are the leading contributor to disability worldwide, with low back pain being the single leading cause of disability in 160 countries.

- Musculoskeletal conditions significantly limit mobility and dexterity, leading to early retirement from work, lower levels of well-being, and reduced ability to participate in society.
- Because of population growth and aging, the number of people living with musculoskeletal conditions and associated functional limitations is rapidly increasing.

The SCL procedure is a robust treatment approach for musculoskeletal injuries, arthritis, sarcopenia (muscle loss), and other conditions affecting bones, muscles, and joints.

Meet David and Roey: How Stem Cells Can Save Knees, Ankles, and Shoulders

One of the most important aspects of being a teenager or young adult is being active physically, going out, participating in sports, and otherwise running around and having as much fun as possible. The older you become, some of this running around might involve working and traveling, too. One of my patients reached out to me concerned about his 16-year-old son, David, who had suffered a right knee meniscal tear during a basketball game. David's friend, who had sustained a similar injury a month prior, had undergone orthopedic surgery and was now immobilized in a brace for 12 weeks and could not play sports for almost a year. David's father inquired about the SCL procedure for his son.

I was glad that he talked to me before they decided to do any surgery. I explained that the stem cells have the unique ability to heal the meniscus cartilage damage, something that contemporary surgical approaches cannot do. More importantly, David's risk and recovery time from the SCL were significantly lower with the SCL procedure, as it does not involve general anesthesia, cutting, stitches, or scars. They agreed to do the SCL.

After the procedure, David got off the table and started to walk with less pain. Just two weeks after the procedure, he was walking with his father on the beach in Cancun during his school break, and within three months he was back to running. David exclaimed to me that the SCL was a life changer, and he couldn't believe that his friend who had undergone the routine surgery was still recovering and unable to play sports.

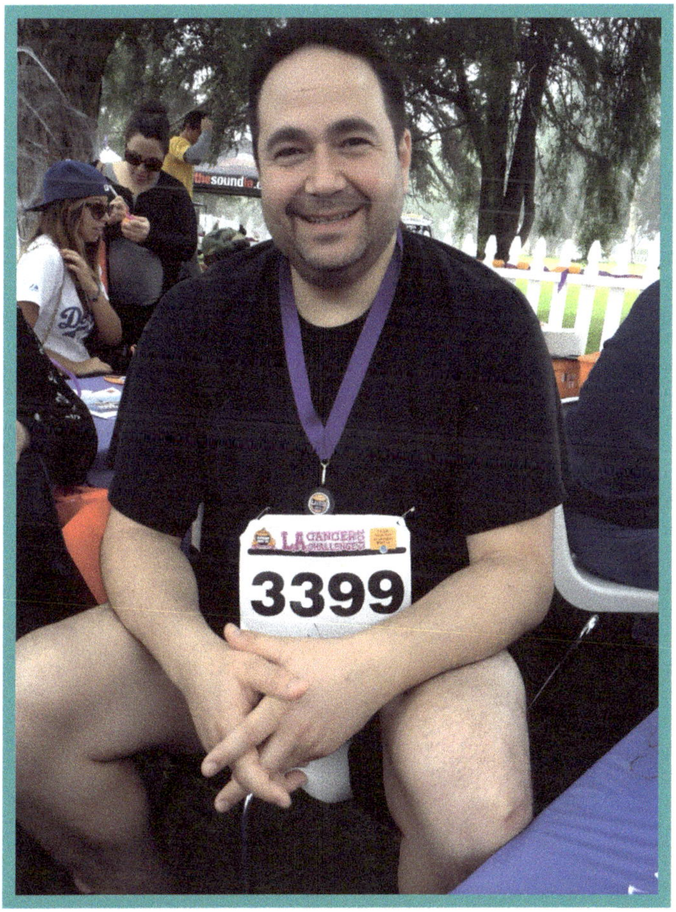

After a doctor told Roey he would need an ankle fusion—a surgery that would have ended his running career, Roey was ecstatic with the life-saving results of my Stem Cell Lift.

Roey, a long-distance runner, was 39 at the time he reached out to me in frustration and fear. Years of running had caused Roey to develop a painful bone cyst on his ankle joint. In addition to near-constant pain in his ankle, Roey's movement was also restricted. Clearly, both conditions were threatening his ability to run. When he had consulted his doctor, Roey was told that he needed surgery to fuse the ankle bones together to avoid a complete collapse of the thinned and weakened bone from the cyst. Ankle fusion is also frequently recommended when end-stage arthritis is diagnosed, the ankle cartilage has worn away, and bone painfully rubs against bone.

This is a big procedure. Ankle fusion (arthrodesis) involves cleaning the worn-out ankle joint and fusing the bones together with screws, plates, and bone grafts. Ankle fusion may relieve pain, but it also greatly limits the ankle's range of motion. The limited mobility can change the patient's gait, which can cause additional wear and tear and ultimately painful arthritis in other joints, such as the hip, knee, and foot. Patients also can spend up to 10 to 12 weeks in a cast. Surgeons may even recommend ankle replacement in some cases. This procedure, known as ankle arthroplasty, replaces the arthritic ankle joint with a metal and plastic prosthesis.

You can imagine how upsetting this news would be to an avid runner: Roey was being told that he would never run again and that he would be limping for the rest of his life!

When we met, I told Roey that I didn't think he had anything to lose by trying to correct the bone cyst with the SCL. In the worst-case scenario, if the stem cell treatment did not correct the problem, he could still have the surgery to fuse the ankle.

Roey agreed.

After concentrating his stem cells from his harvested fat cells, I gently aspirated the fluid that had built up around the cyst. Then I injected his stem cells using the SCL method.

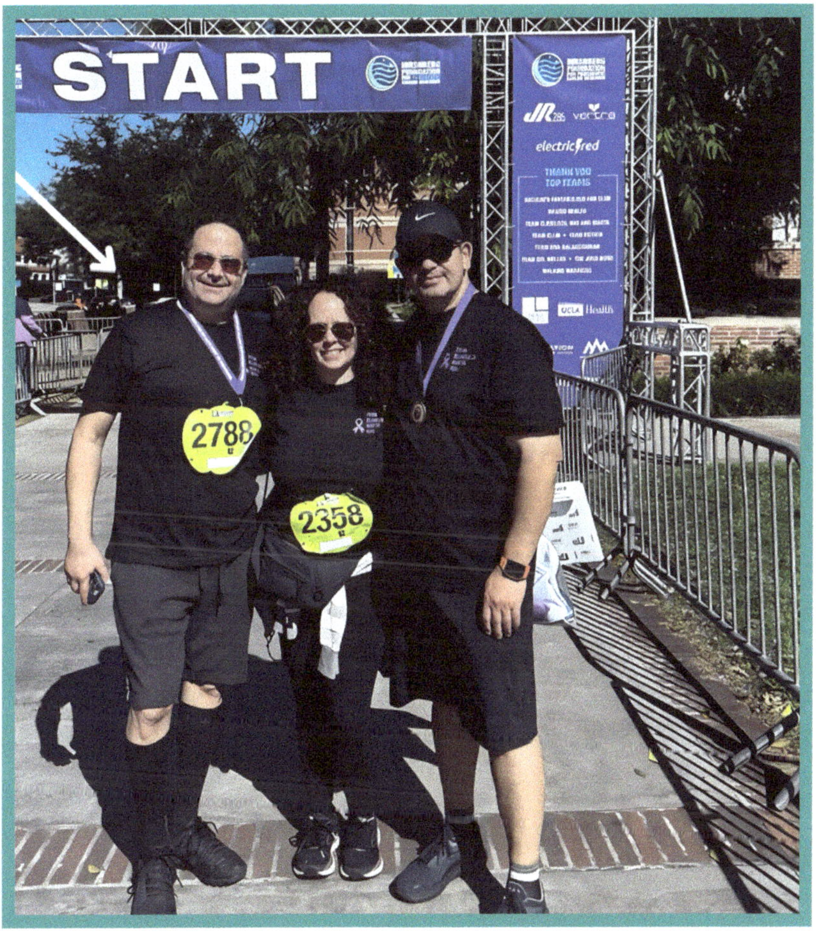

Roey will be forever grateful for the SCL, which has not only restored his ability to walk but also to run without pain.

Six weeks later, x-rays showed not only that the cyst was gone but that the ankle had healed. Roey was soon running again and still is to this day.

Treating My Own Shoulder

I am very active and play a number of sports, and like many a middle-aged athlete, eventually I got a muscle injury, tearing my rotator cuff.

At first, I tried conservative treatments, including physical therapy and noninvasive treatments such as low-level red light laser, PEMF, and AVACEN therapy—but without improvement. As my pain got progressively worse, my range of motion became increasingly limited. At night, I could not find a comfortable position and I could not sleep due to the pain. I then decided to inject platelet-rich plasma (PRP) into the shoulder in hopes of getting some relief.

Despite two PRP injections two weeks apart, however, my shoulder was not feeling any better. At this point I decided to have the SCL procedure to heal my shoulder. This was a bit of a challenge, as I am slim, and I was going to carry out the procedure on myself. Thankfully, I have a very capable, experienced, and kind staff who helped me. I numbed the area on my trunk to take the fat, harvested the fat, and concentrated the stem cells. Within 48 hours of injecting my stem cells into my shoulder, I felt significant relief. In two weeks I felt much better, and by three months I had regained my full range of motion. I continued to see improvement—even six months out.

What Is PRP?

Platelets found in the circulating blood in our veins are tasked with stopping bleeding and signaling the body to heal the injured tissue. Platelets contain wound-healing factors. A blood draw is carried out and the blood is put in a special tube and centrifuged to separate the red blood cells from the platelets. The albumin-rich protein in the liquid part of the blood is called plasma. The concentrated platelets in the plasma are drawn up into a syringe and injected into the tissue to induce healing. PRP therapy can be used alone or with stem cells to enhance the regenerative effect.

If you or a loved one is suffering from any muscle, tendon, cartilage, or joint pain or injury, or even a longstanding condition (such as bone-on-bone arthritis, meniscus tear, and tendonitis), I recommend exploring the option of stem cell therapy before you undergo invasive surgery. The stem cell alternative may help improve the quality of your life, without the pain, risks, and lengthy recovery of a surgery.

“Aging is not a disease. It is a natural process of life. However, there are many ways to delay the process and improve the quality of life through the years. Stem cell therapy plays a key role in making aging more pleasant, enjoyable, and graceful.”

—DR. NATHAN NEWMAN

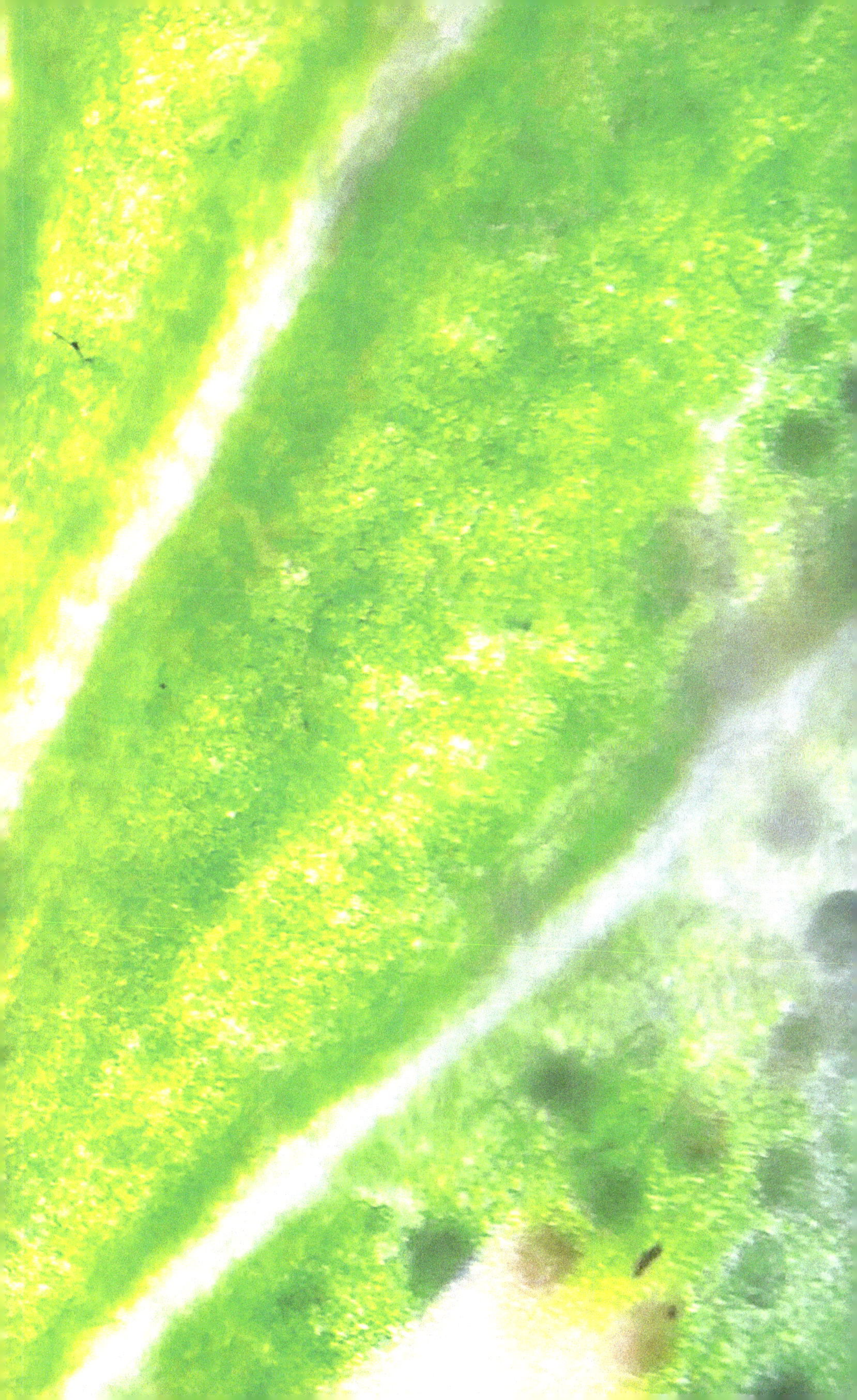

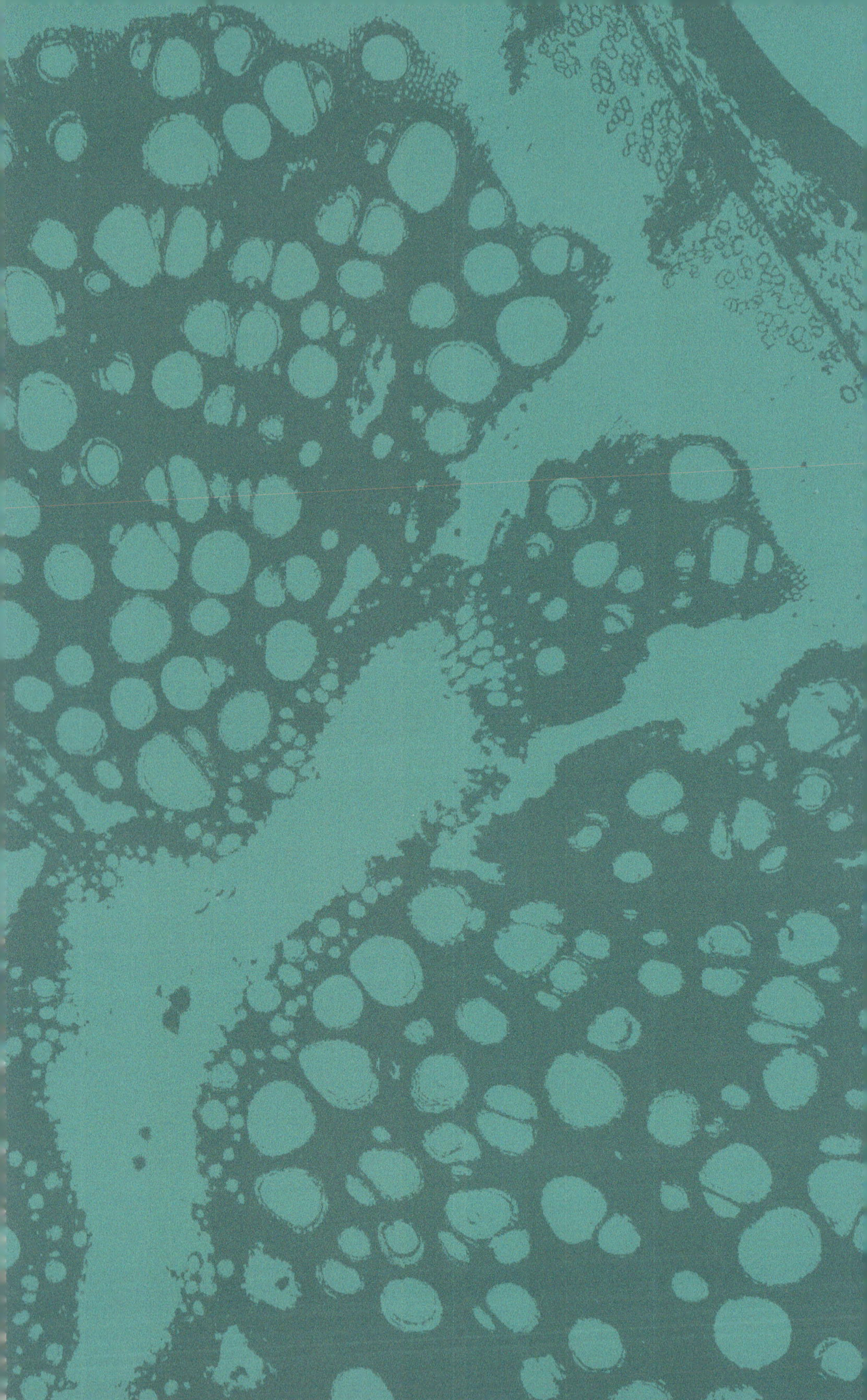

7

How the Stem Cell Lift Restores and Rejuvenates Appearance

As I mentioned earlier in the book, my mission is not about stopping or reversing the aging process; rather, I think about aging from a different point—an earlier point. When women and men come to me for the Stem Cell Lift to reduce the effects of aging—wrinkles, sagging skin, discoloration of the skin, and loss of facial volume and bone structure—I explain that I don't want to *change* their appearance, I want to *restore* their natural beauty and return them to a place where they feel like their best selves. In fact, many of my patients tell me after they've received the procedure that they feel like they look better than they did when they were younger!

To capture the sense of the overall effect of the SCL, I like to use the metaphor of transforming a raisin back into a grape. Instead of cutting and pulling, I'm filling, rejuvenating, and lifting. I'm not changing the integrity of your face or neck; I am giving it back what it has lost as a result of aging—that quality of vitality that we associate with youth. As we age, we lose volume from atrophy of fat, muscles, and bone structures; we also lose skin integrity as the skin thins and becomes inelastic. This is why the skin begins to droop and wrinkle, giving us a tired and drawn appearance. The procedure harnesses the regenerative powers of your own stem cells to sculpt the tissues in 3D, creating an appealing symmetry and restoring the proper proportions to your entire face. The stem cells bring back a youthful, healthy glow by enhancing the skin's volume, collagen structure, blood flow, and elasticity in the face, neck, chest, hands, and other areas. Of course, there is no one cause of aging—the pace at which one ages is related to a unique combination of genetic factors, environmental stress, and lifestyle, including nutrition, frequency of physical exercise, amount and quality of sleep, and whether one engages in energy-depleting habits such as smoking and excessive drinking of alcohol.

Meet Carmen: Restoring a Youthful Glow

Feeling frustrated, Carmen came to see me. She said that over the past few years, her skin had lost its vitality and she'd developed dark circles beneath her eyes. When I described the Stem Cell Lift procedure, she jumped at the chance to pursue a new way to address her concerns.

Take a look at the before and after photos of Carmen.

In the before photo, her skin looks uneven and she has dark-appearing circles under her eyes. In the after photo, the quality of her skin looks smoother, the pigmentation on her cheekbones has all but disappeared, and her eyes look less puffy. Just three months after

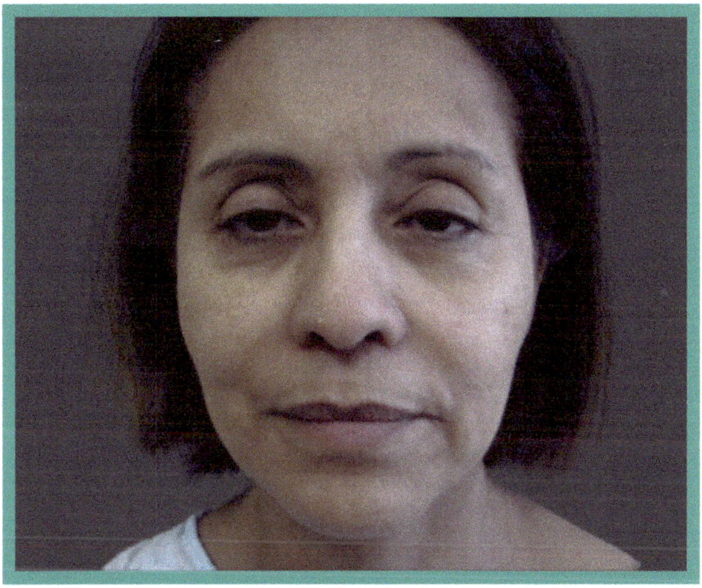

Before

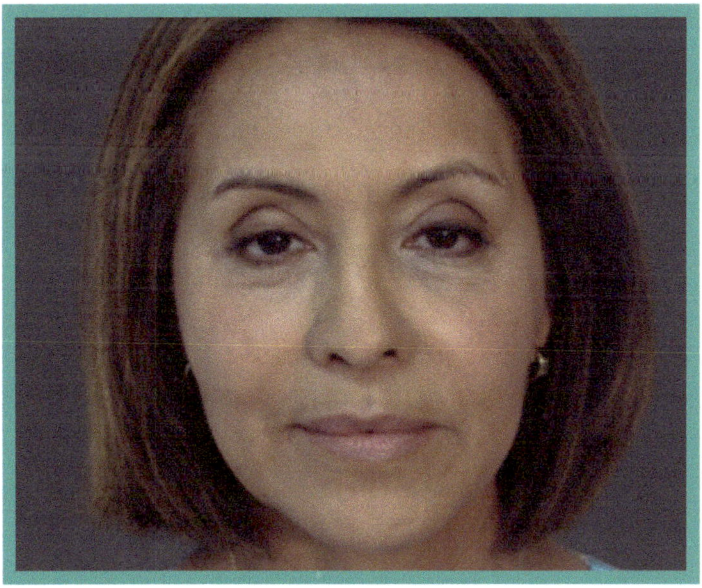

After one year

Carmen looks rejuvenated, youthful, and refreshed after my exclusive Stem Cell Lift.

a SCL treatment, the injected stem cells addressed the sagging and discoloration, enhancing the quality of her skin, and replenished the "holes" to restore volume.

> I don't want to *change* a patient's appearance, I want to *restore* their natural beauty and return them to a place where they feel like their best selves. In fact, many of my patients tell me after they've received the SCL treatment that they feel like they look better than they did when they were younger!

People of all ages can benefit from the SCL procedure. In other words, you don't have to wait until you're in your 50s or 60s to benefit from stem cell treatment. Compared to artificial fillers and implants, the SCL is a much more natural and wholesome approach to feeling and looking younger. Take a look at this quite youthful woman in her early 40s.

How the Stem Cell Lift Differs from the Traditional Facelift

Before developing the Stem Cell Lift procedure, when I was performing more traditional cutting and pulling facelifts, I noticed that although my facelift patients initially looked good, over the course of a few years they appeared older. It became clear to me after observing these changes that although the two-dimensional (2D) traditional facelift was tightening the skin, the process of cutting and pulling the skin was causing the healthy tissues underneath the skin to scar, lose their blood flow, and make the skin thin and crepey. I noticed when the skin was pulled tight over the bony structures, it made the person look hollowed, skeletonized, and therefore older. The use of fillers and even fat grafting for the cheeks or other specific areas only exaggerated this undesirable appearance.

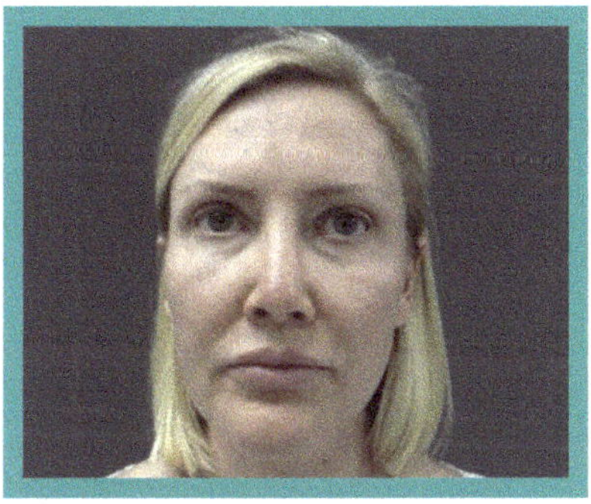

Before

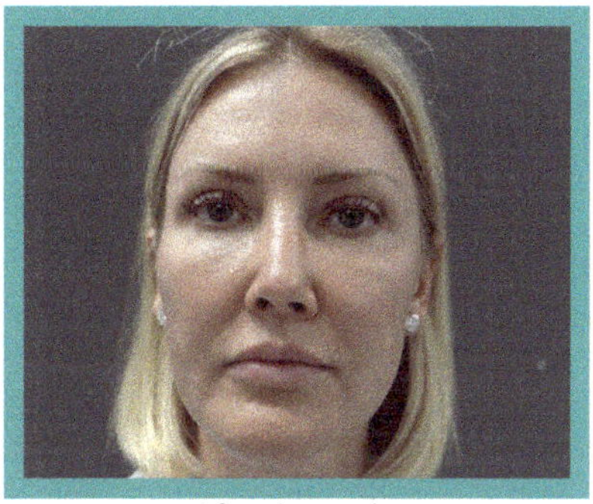

After six months

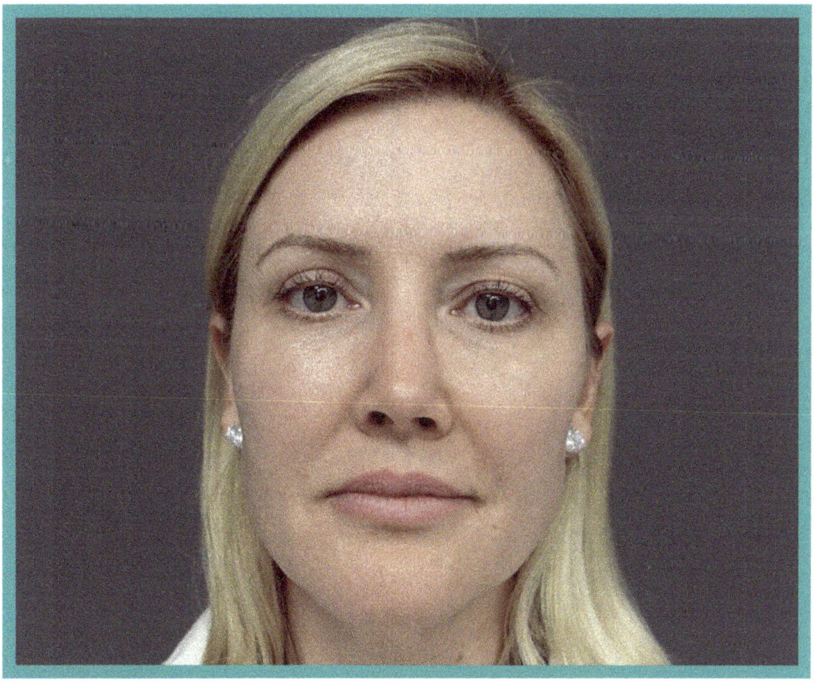

After one year

This patient continues to see youthful improvements one year after her SCL.

When I began using my procedure, the results were remarkably different. My patients who had received the stem cell–enriched fat injections were looking *even better* with time. Their skin was plumper, more elastic, smoother, and toned, and it had a youthful glow. As I perfected my SCL procedure and saw the dramatic and rapid improvement in my patients' appearance, I switched from cutting and pulling with a scalpel and sutures to rejuvenating and restoring the tissues with my patients' own stem cells. With the SCL procedure I can sculpt the face three-dimensionally to achieve the desired youthful, healthy, and aesthetic proportions. At the same time, the stem cells restore the collagen and elastin scaffolding, the microvasculature, and the volume, naturally becoming part of the tissues without changing normal vectors of facial movement and animation.

The difference between my approach to cosmetic enhancement and the common facelift surgery is dramatic and consequential. This is because tighter does not make younger. Again, think of the idea of taking a grape and turning it into a raisin; this is how skin ages. If I were to pull the wrinkled surface of the raisin, I don't get the grape back—but if I inject stem cells into the raisin, it restores the grape. The SCL achieves beautiful, youthful results with no cutting of the skin, no use of general anesthesia, and virtually no risk of bleeding, nerve damage, or scarring. Patients who undergo treatment walk out of my office and return to their daily lives almost immediately. The initial swelling and any bruising that may occur usually resolves within two weeks and within three months my patients enjoy a permanent enhancement to their face, neck, and hands.

When you understand the difference between the three-dimensional SCL and the traditional two-dimensional facelift method, you are able to make fully informed decisions. In a two-dimensional procedure, long cuts are made into the skin on the sides of the face and then pulled tight to address the sagging and wrinkling. In order to get the "lift," the skin may be pulled too tight at times. Not only does this stretching action often look too tight, giving that "windblown in a tunnel" look, but it also reduces the natural movement of the facial muscles. This is when women and men who have "had work done" look as if they can't smile or they've lost their facial expressions.

When I use the Stem Cell Lift procedure, replenishing the underlying tissue with the stem cells, I am restoring the natural contour of your face, using the natural vectors that are already in place. By maintaining your natural vectors, my procedure enables you to maintain your smile lines, your eye crinkles, and the movement of your cheekbones when you speak. Again, this is about preserving your natural look. A traditional two-dimensional facelift does not maintain your natural vectors, which is why men and women tend to look altered and odd, especially when making facial expressions.

The SCL procedure is not only a more comprehensive approach to achieving a rejuvenated look but also significantly safer and far superior to the traditional facelift.

Another important advantage of my procedure over traditional facelift and plastic surgery is that the SCL addresses the entire face in one procedure and without all the risks, complications, recovery time, pain, and costs associated with traditional plastic surgery. Specifically, a "facelift" is a neck and lower facelift procedure. To address the midface, forehead, upper and lower eyelids, lips, chin, jawline, earlobes, and nose would each require a separate scarring procedure and technique, while the SCL alone replaces all of these nine procedures. In addition, the SCL procedure can also address the décolleté (chest) and the back of the hands simultaneously, making it not only a more comprehensive approach to achieving a rejuvenated look but also significantly safer and far superior to the traditional facelift.

Table 1: The traditional 2D facelift vs. the 3D Stem Cell Lift

TRADITIONAL FACELIFT	STEM CELL LIFT
Unnatural results (pulled and distorted)	Natural results (proportional and youthful)
May look different	Look the same but better
Difficult, painful, and long recovery time	Easy and short recovery time
Lasts from 2 to 10 years	Permanent improvement lasting 10+ years as stem cells replace old cells
General anesthesia risks (including death)	No general anesthesia risks
Cutting skin and scarring	No cutting, no scars
Stitches	No stitches
Increased risk of complications (e.g., nerve damage, bleeding, infection, allergic reaction)	Minimized risk of complications (e.g., nerve damage, bleeding, infection, allergic reaction)
May use foreign materials (e.g., sutures, implants)	Uses your own fat and stem cells
Long and painful recovery requiring pain medications	Short recovery from swelling and soreness
Causes skin to thin	Improves skin texture and tone
Can result in decreased sensation or tingling (pins and needles) in the skin	Normal sensation
Weeks to recover	Minimal downtime (can resume regular activities the next day)
Lengthy procedure time	Fast procedure
Need separate procedures for each area, increasing risk, cost, procedure time, and recovery	Can combine eight or more procedures simultaneously with no scars and minimal added risk, cost, procedure time, and recovery time

TRADITIONAL FACELIFT	STEM CELL LIFT
Addresses only the lower face and neck. Different surgical procedures are needed to address different areas of the face: • Forehead lift • Brow lift • Blepharoplasty • Midface lift • Face lift • Neck lift • Rhinoplasty • Lip lift • Chin augmentation (implant) • Cheek implants	Treats entire face, neck, and hands with a mini-liposuction on the body as a bonus. Examples of areas that can be improved: • Forehead • Temples • Eyes • Nose • Lips • Mid-face (cheeks and laugh lines) • Lateral face • Lower face (jowls) • Jawline • Chin • Earlobes • Neck • Hands

Advantages of the Stem Cell Lift over Fillers

While many cosmetic products promise such rejuvenating results, they cannot approximate the effects of the stem cells, which, by their very nature, adhere to the underlying tissue and build it back. Traditional fillers and other cosmetic products that promise to rejuvenate do not regenerate. This is an important distinction. Stem cells give the body the capacity to build back the tissues that are typically lost as people age. The stem cells work with the body to repair, restore, and rejuvenate, which is why I tell patients that with the SCL they will rediscover the best version of themselves. Although SCL technically may be used merely to volumize tissues in a similar way to an injectable filler, using a person's own fat-derived stem cells is entirely different from using a synthetic substance. Most of the cosmetic fillers used today contain hyaluronic acid (HA) or calcium hydroxylapatite (CaHA). Injecting the skin around the lips, eyes, or cheekbones with a typical filler doesn't correct or address what's missing underneath the skin; it simply fills the space with a temporary substance that is static and inert and cannot become part of dynamic and living tissues. Because of these factors, fillers often result in an unnatural appearance. In contrast, the SCL offers women and men a natural look that enhances their appearance from the inside out.

Because of its small particle size, it takes a lot of synthetic filler to volumize the tissues, making people look puffy or lumpy. One syringe of stem cell–enriched fat cells is approximately 5 to 10 syringes of other fillers in terms of volumization. When you fill in too much, a person can look deformed and not proportional. The goal of natural restoration is missed. Moreover, cosmetic enhancement is not about perfection—far from it. We are not symmetrical. One side of your face does not perfectly mirror the other side. Your bone and fat on one side of your face are not exactly the same as the other. During cosmetic enhancement and rejuvenation, we address this asymmetry with a focus on maintaining a natural and balanced look. Your beauty is encapsulated in your uniqueness and relative symmetrical proportions. Therefore, it is important to follow the vectors of the original you. Years of experience in restoring natural-looking, youthful, and healthy proportions has been the blueprint for my success.

Your beauty is encapsulated in your uniqueness and relative symmetrical proportions. Therefore, it is important to follow the vectors of the original you. Years of experience in restoring natural-looking, youthful, and healthy proportions has been the blueprint for my success.

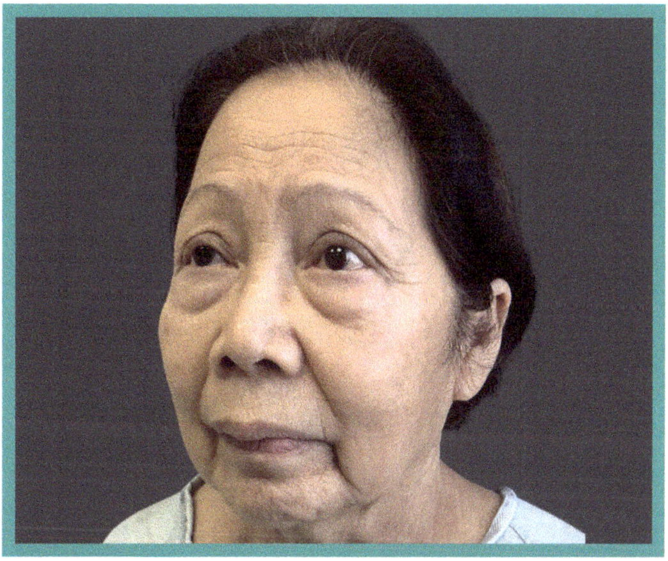

Before

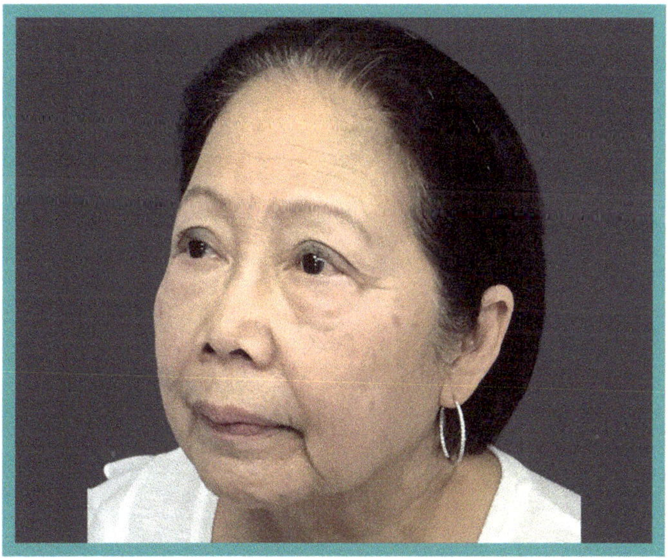

After one year

Many of my patients are surprised to learn that the SCL can be used instead of the traditional lower blepharoplasty. Rather than cutting out skin and fat, which can leave the under-eye area looking hollow and aged, I use my innovative SCL to restore the youthful appearance without cutting.

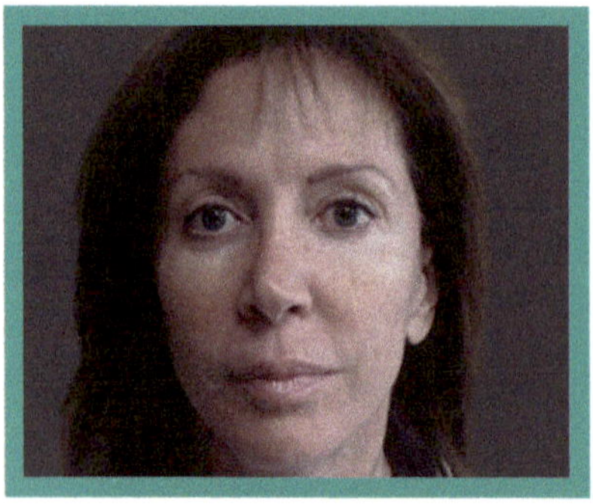

Before

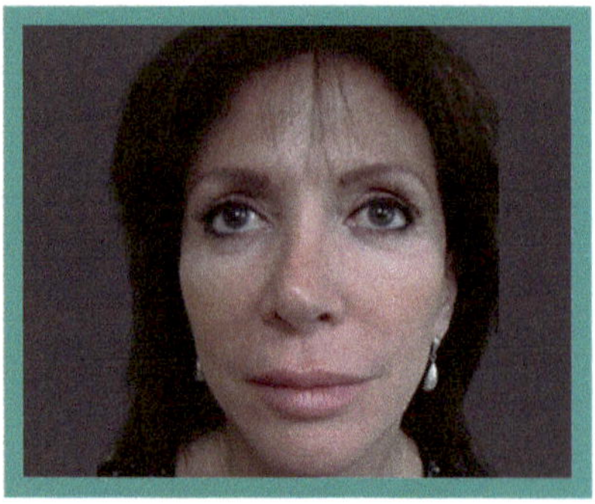

After two years

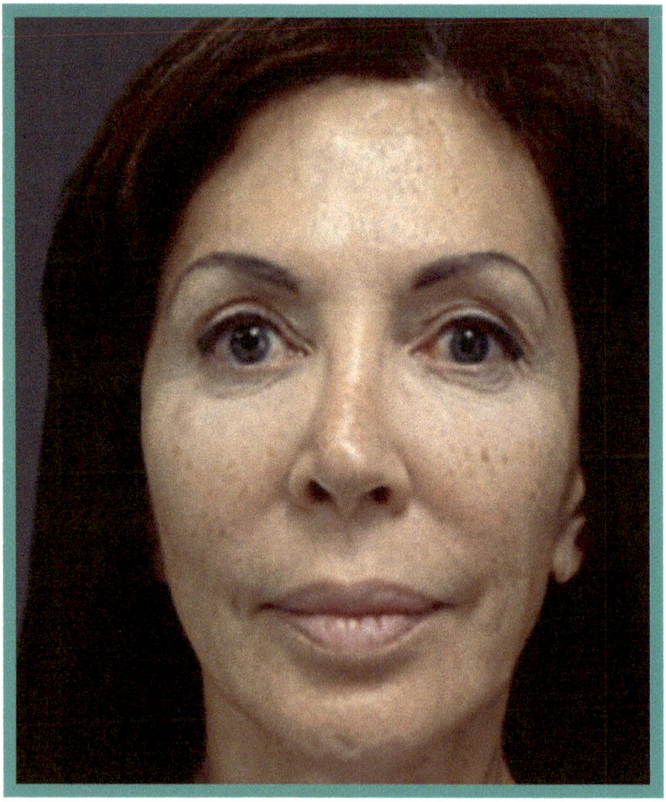

After 12 years

This news reporter opted to have the SCL procedure after a traditional facelift left her feeling hollow and appearing disproportional. Using stem cells from her own fat, I subtly sculpted the contours of her face, restoring her natural, youthful appearance.

Treating Hands with Stem Cells

A tell-tale sign of a woman's age is her hands. As mentioned, one of the benefits of the SCL is that I can, in one procedure, address the face, neck, chest, and hands and rejuvenate all the areas most associated with looking aged, older, and tired.

Stem Cells for Breast and Buttocks Enhancement

I also use the Stem Cell Lift to shape or lift the breasts and buttocks. Given the risks associated with silicone implants and the actual risks of going under the knife and general anesthesia, many women today are seeking a more natural, safer alternative to enhance their breasts and buttocks. Instead of undergoing costly surgery, which always

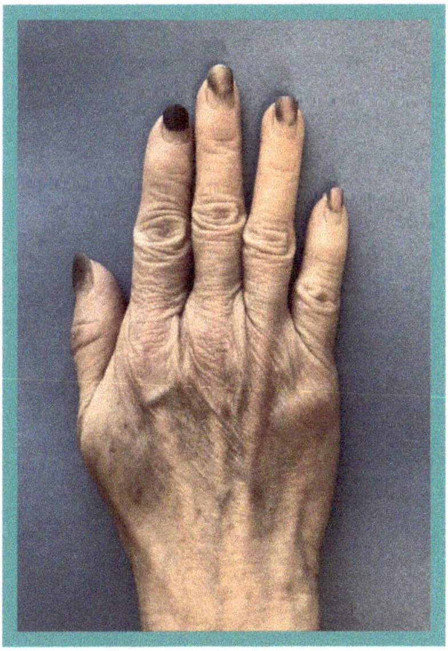

Before

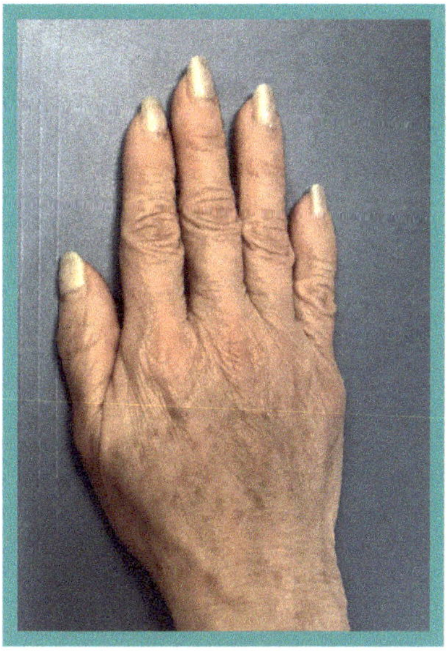

After four months

Don't let your hands give away your age. Many patients that undergo the SCL opt to have their hands treated with stem cells as well. The SCL works to restore volume while improving skin quality.

entails risks of anesthesia and long recuperation, the SCL offers a noninvasive alternative way to regain plumpness to the buttocks, lift the breasts to their youthful shape, and restore women's confidence in their overall physique.

Breast Enhancement

The SCL procedure offers a natural and innovative way to enhance the breasts, providing enough volume to potentially increase the size by one cup. Using your own fat, rich in regenerative stem cells, this technique not only adds fullness and shape to the breasts but also contours other areas of the body through gentle fat harvesting. The result is a dual benefit: a natural-looking enhancement and improved body proportions. Since no implants are used, the risks associated with foreign materials, such as rupture, rejection, contraction scarring, or the need for surgery to replace the implant, are eliminated. The recovery is also much easier and faster, with almost no restrictions on daily activities immediately after the procedure. The injected fat also helps improve imaging of the breast glands during routine exams. This permanent yet natural enhancement will last for years.

Buttocks Enhancement

The SCL procedure is a natural and effective option for enhancing the buttocks, improving volume, shape, and contour. By using your own fat, enriched with your own regenerative stem cells, I remove excess fat from the lower back, lateral thighs, inner thighs, and the "banana folds" under the buttocks to enhance the shape and proportions of the buttocks and the areas around it. I then use this stem cell–enriched fat to lift and shape the buttocks, enhancing your overall silhouette. Since no synthetic implants are used, the risks associated with foreign materials, such as infection or displacement, are avoided. There are no scars, the recovery is easier than that for implants, and the buttocks feel and look natural.

As you will see in the forthcoming chapters, my journey into stem cell technology continued. Although I continue to use the SCL procedure with great success, treating thousands of patients each year, I have also delved into the power of stem cell language and how we decipher it in the laboratory to create cell-free off-the-shelf products to make this technology available to all.

PART III

The New Frontier of Stem Cell Technology

> *“Stem cell technology, to me, is a gift of the present and the promise of the near future.”*
>
> —DR. NATHAN NEWMAN

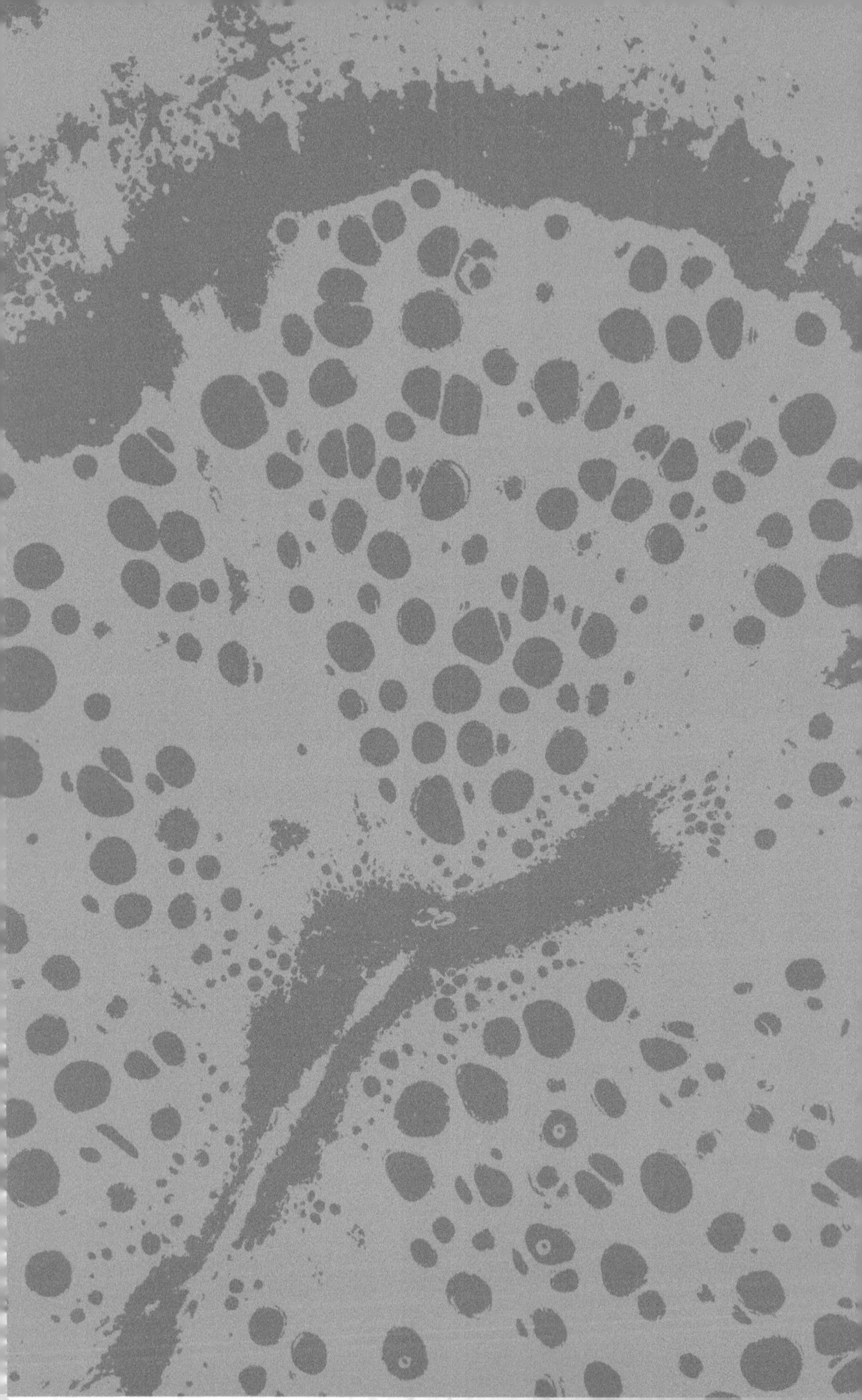

8

Discovering the Language of Stem Cells

My father, my brother, and other great mentors of mine instilled in me the importance and power of observation, which has helped lead me to innovation and discovery. In observing the dramatic and rapid skin improvements in my SCL patients, I began to question the underlying mechanisms that produced such significant positive effects. In general, cellular changes take a few months to become apparent in the body. With stem cells I was seeing changes within a few days of injecting them into a patient's tissues.

Meet Helaine: Skin Improvement in Just Four Weeks

Helaine is a good example of how quickly the skin improves after the Stem Cell Lift. Consider the photo of Helaine before treatment, and then just one month after.

I hypothesized that these changes were being caused by something the cells were *producing*—not simply the presence of the stem cells themselves. The scientist in me became curious as to what this might be and inspired me to research stem cells in the laboratory. Thanks to the vision and support of my wife, I opened my first lab in my Beverly Hills medical institute and soon after hired my first stem cell scientist to study what stem cells produce. This small lab allowed me to continue to research stem cells and create that wonderful synergy between clinic practice and ongoing research, which had always been a dream of mine. This led me to investigate the world of stem cell language and cellular communication. Just like when I realized many practitioners were throwing away the "gold" in the fat when they began retrieving stem cells from adipose tissue, I had the sense that something similar was going on—I was once again the maverick challenging the status quo.

Soon we learned that stem cells communicate and signal each other and other cells through proteins and chemicals that they produce. The chemical language that the cells secrete to communicate with other cells is called the secretome, and its composition changes based on the environment the cells are in. This was consistent with my clinical experience: a specific cellular response is based on the cellular environment in which it takes place. These results pointed me in an interesting direction: to the importance of the paracrine effect, or how cells communicate back and forth through these secretory factors. This was a huge moment for me. Just as the stem cells had been overlooked in the clinic, the beneficial secretory factors produced

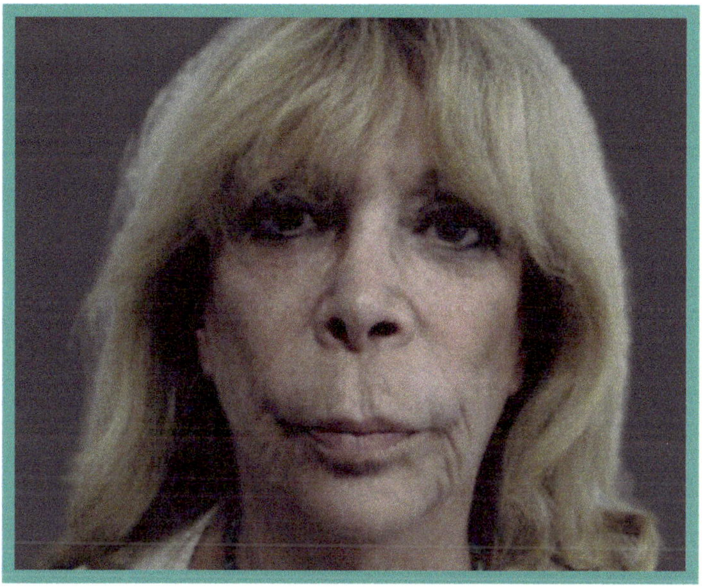

Before

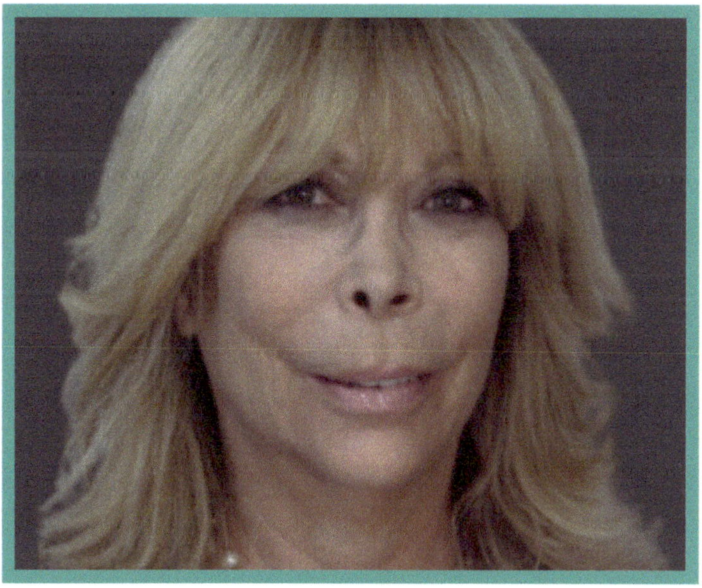

After one month

Just four weeks after her SCL, Helaine is constantly getting comments like "You look so rested, did you just come back from vacation?"

by the stem cells were being overlooked by scientists. Other scientists focused only on the stem cells they grew in the lab, regarding the liquid growth media in which the cells developed as waste. From seeing the rapid effects of stem cells in the clinic, I realized the potential of the secretory factors being produced in the cell culture media. What if we used this broth to treat tissues?

I started testing this theory on wounds with surprisingly good results. I also observed improvement in the skin wounds and soon started testing it on intact skin. In a matter of a few weeks, I saw the sun-damaged, wrinkled skin improve substantially.

Along with treating my cosmetic patients with the stem cell procedure, I also began to develop topical serums, always trying to honor the natural beauty of my myriad patients. Part of my motivation to create such products was to help not only my patients, but also anyone who could not come to see me in person in California. I wanted to raise awareness of this new paradigm of natural intelligence and make the innovative stem cell technology available to as many people as possible so that they, too, could benefit from the healing properties of stem cells. Also, I wanted to share my growing understanding of the power of stem cells with other physicians, hoping to open their eyes and minds to these remarkable findings, which fascinated me as a physician and a scientist. In order to promote these ideas, I continued to write in scientific journals and in medical books, present at conferences, and tirelessly contribute and advance the professional discussion about the enormous potential of stem cells to heal and prevent disease.

We were also looking at how to get the best stem cells for clinical use. Did it make a difference where on the body the cells were harvested from? Again, I was looking at how the cell signaling played a role and if the stem cells differed based on body region. The results from this study, published in 2019, showed that the "proliferation and viability" of the stem cells harvested from different areas of the body (abdomen, flanks, and thighs, specifically) were similar.[1]

What Are the Stem Cells Secreting?

Along with my dedicated team of scientists, I began looking at the factors that the stem cells were secreting. Stem cells release what we call "secretory factors," including growth factors, cytokines, chemokines, peptides, proteins, small molecules, and exosomes. Together these molecules help to control intercellular communication and interactions in all biological systems, especially the immune system. I knew from the research at the time that scientists were looking at the potential therapeutic effects of isolated secretory factors. But just as I had zeroed in on preserving the stem cells in the fat, I now wanted to isolate the environmental milieu of the stem cells—the secretome—and keep it intact.

Early uses of stem cells for therapeutic purposes had not gone as planned due to a lack of understanding of the nature of stem cells and how to control their pathways for healing. Many physicians still thought that stem cells injected or introduced directly into a damaged or diseased area of the body were responsible for the positive healing effects. In one now-infamous case, a California woman in her 60s underwent a procedure in which stem cells were injected into her eyelids in order to give her a more youthful appearance. Three months after the procedure, she was experiencing inordinate pain and a clicking sound in her eye.

The woman then reached out to another surgeon, who regrettably had to tell the woman that the stem cells had grown bone in her eyelid. Following a lengthy surgery in which the doctor removed small pieces of bone from her eyelid and the surrounding tissue, the woman began to recover. The clicks the woman had heard were a result of the bone fragments pushing against one another.

This is a powerful example of the misinformation around stem cells and triggered the false belief that stem cells are dangerous. In this woman's case, the stem cells were injected with calcium hydroxyapatite filler, and the calcium-rich filler signaled the stem cells to differentiate toward and create bonelike structures. They were told by their environment to make bone, and so they did. Had the calcium-rich filler been replaced by another filler—or better yet, had no other product been injected with the cells—no bone would have formed in this patient's eyelid.

I have spent years lecturing and explaining that the cells actually did what they were supposed to do. This terrible example shows both the power of stem cells and their potential based on their environment. Because of their innate capacity to differentiate and take on the characteristics of the cells where they are introduced, stem cells will do as they're told, so to speak. In the woman's case, the stem cells injected into her eyelid predictably grew bone. Had the doctor really wanted to grow bone in the woman's eyelid? No. But what he didn't understand at the time was how best to use stem cells: their power comes not through injection directly, but rather through the paracrine effect, which enables the stem cells and their secretomes to target the area in need indirectly. Indeed, it's this cell-to-cell dialogue through their secretomes that actually directs the stem cells. And this was an important clue that I had begun to follow.

The Paracrine Effect

So what is this mysterious paracrine effect? Our bodies rely on cell signaling for development, growth (cell division), excretion, and repair of damage to cells, tissues, or organs. There are several different types of cell-signaling systems, including endocrine (hormones secreted through the blood or circulatory system), exocrine (via ducts through sweat glands, for example), and paracrine. Paracrine signaling is a form of cell-to-cell communication in which a cell produces a signal to induce changes in nearby cells, altering their behavior or triggering differentiation.

Early research on the significance of the paracrine effect focused on its potential for regenerative medicine as a whole and in particular its role in stem cell communication (signaling). Scientists began seeing evidence of paracrine action in many cardiovascular studies. Given that coronary artery disease and heart failure are leading causes of death worldwide, these findings were heartening. Researchers pointed to how paracrine effects contribute to the improvement of cardiac function following tissue damage by targeting inflammation, fibrosis, apoptosis, growth of new blood cells, and repair of the heart muscle itself, similar to the results I was seeing with the SCL in the clinic when treating muscle injury or performing reconstructive therapy.

Again, the therapeutic effects of stem cells are regulated by three main mechanisms:

- Migration to site of injury
- Differentiation into various cell types that can engraft to the damaged tissue
- Secretion of bioactive factors

But until recently, these mechanisms were isolated from the paracrine effect. I was intrigued by the implications related to the protective and regenerative effects of different stem cell therapies. With this information, I began to work with different types of cells in the laboratory setting. I wanted to understand what the cells were doing and what they were producing. I also wanted to discern how best to create different environments for cell growth to produce the outcomes we were looking for. I knew that the stimuli in any micro-environment would affect the composition of the secretory factors. And third, I wanted to understand best how to utilize and apply the power of the secretome, the set of molecules and biological factors that are secreted by cells into the extracellular space. I knew that I could produce the secretome in my lab, which meant I could harness it for clinical use.

If I wanted to stimulate hair growth, which cultured medium would work best? What combination of plant and human stem cells would work best?

If I wanted to stimulate regrowth of collagen and improve the elasticity of the skin, what combination of factors should I use?

If a wound was not healing properly, what combination of stem cell factors could help strengthen the immune response to enable expedited and full repair of the wound?

By studying the quantities and types of stem cell–secreted factors and, most importantly, designing the micro-environment where these factors get "seeded," I was able to do what other researchers had not yet been able to do: take advantage of the incredible plasticity of stem cells through the paracrine mechanism and control its secretome to produce a reliable, predictable, and reproducible set of directions that can be used on the body. I was after the entire direction found in the secretome (i.e., the paracrine factors secreted from the stem cells), not just an isolated molecule or component of the secretome, such as exosomes.

By studying the quantities and types of stem cell–secreted factors and, most importantly, designing the micro-environment where these factors get "seeded," I was able to do what other researchers had not yet been able to do.

Even today, with the growing popularity of using exosomes to repair and rejuvenate the skin, for example, many are still missing the point. While exosomes contain numerous growth factors and are important mediators of paracrine signaling and intercellular communication, their current uses do not take into account the entirety of the secretome. Indeed, exosomes represent only one component of the necessary secretory factors of stem cells. My wholistic approach grows, collects, and utilizes the whole of the secretome, including exosomes, which enables me not only to direct the purpose of the stem cell language (i.e., the secretome in its cultured media) but also to create a much more powerful effect.

> I don't try to manipulate or interfere with the natural intelligence of the body. I always try to follow and assist nature, not work against it.

I often use the analogy of grandma's healing chicken soup when I explain the difference between exosomes and secretome. The exosomes are only one ingredient in the soup, and thus much less effective by themselves. The soup as a whole—that is, exosomes, peptides, proteins, and all of the other secretory factors combined—is organically and synergistically much more potent and therapeutic. Current exosome therapy is both inexact and incomplete in its impact because, in order to extract the exosomes from the secretome in which they are produced, the laboratory processes the product, throwing out the highly valuable soup of the cellular language. In addition, the exosome process can also include the addition of artificial factors meant to increase the impact of the exosomes. In contrast, I don't try to manipulate or interfere with the natural intelligence of the body. I always try to follow and assist nature, not work against it.

Back in my lab, we began to develop two things: an array of unique combinations of secretory factors and a process that we could use reliably to direct and predict the effects of the various secretomes. This was not a linear process; as we were discovering the importance of this unique set of directions being secreted by the stem cells, what we now call the Consortia Factors (CFx), we went through a lot of trial and error. For instance, I didn't know how specific plant cells would interact with one another or with human-derived stem cells. My team and I tested many different cells and, lo and behold, we began to see patterns emerging in our data with certain stem cell combinations. We also experimented with cell cultures, one of the most common methods to create a controlled environment in a laboratory setting. Cell culture techniques are used to grow and maintain cells of various types, including stem cells. However, one of the challenges to this method is always the unwitting introduction of foreign matter that could undermine results. Therefore, my team and I developed innovative methods and products to allow us to grow the cells free of animal sources, which could harbor disease or cause adverse reactions and toxic chemicals that, in turn, might harm the cells in the lab or my patients in the clinic.

As we began looking at how plant stem cells and human stem cells interacted in certain situations or environments, my research team and I were able to directly mentor and guide these interactions: we could choose certain plant stem cells to interact with human stem cells and track their results. This wasn't a process that we had mapped out, but as we began to get results, we became more deliberate and mindful, developing processes that were defined for each Consortia Factor.

We discovered we could bottle these factors and then apply them to the skin. And what we saw was amazing: we observed dramatic effects beyond the local effect—this was clear evidence of the paracrine feedback effect. We began testing various CFx to formulate topical, inhalant, ingestible, or injectable medicinal products for specific purposes, such as skin regeneration, hair growth, skin burns, lung problems, cartilage repair, and bone repair.

But again, the specific products were not as important as the whole platform: with this technology (which included my approach to harvesting stem cells, creating and utilizing the CFx), I could imagine developing thousands of products to address thousands of conditions and issues. “What’s the problem? Let’s create a product to fix it!” There’s no limit to using stem cell technology in this way!

My team, which I led alongside our chief scientific officer, Dodanim Talavera-Adame, MD, PhD, decided to call this novel biotechnology process *stem cell mentoring* because the way in which we direct the growth of various stem cell factors is similar to the concept of mentoring: with our unique process (i.e., the platform), we help guide the stem cells. Our platform allows us to grow any human or plant stem cell and direct it to create a specific secretome-rich cultured media (the CFx). We had two goals in mind: to better direct the CFx for desired results and to establish a reliable and reproducible process for directing those results. Not only is this biotechnological process completely original, it’s also been awarded a patent.

Patenting Our Mentoring Process

Together with my interdisciplinary team of medical doctors and scientists specializing in stem cell biotechnology, we developed a patent for this revolutionary stem cell technology process. In late 2022, we received notification that our patent, entitled “System and Method for the Production, Formulation, and Use of Conditioned Media, Cultured Cells, and the Factors Included Therein,” had been issued. We were ecstatic! The patent and all that it represents—more than two decades of hard work and dedication, research, and clinical experimentation and data collection with my team had come to fruition.

The patent solidified the recognition of our research and development and the credibility of our innovation.

This innovative platform technology allows renewable, green, sustainable culturing of any stem cell or combinations of cells to produce unique sets of cultured media, secretory factors, peptides, and exosomes: Consortia Factors. These profiles refer to the patent’s innovative method of "figuring out the language of the cells" that promotes and enhances the anti-inflammatory, regenerative, rejuvenating, or pro-healing cascade within the targeted tissues of the body. These key ingredients are then used to formulate clean, organic, and biobased solutions, including:

- Cosmetics for skin, hair, and nails
- Compounded, over-the-counter (OTC) medications, including topical pain relievers, anti-inflammatories, and other analgesics
- Topical and injectable pharmaceutical products that advance the treatment of a wide variety of medical conditions
- Inhalants for respiratory issues
- Oral superfoods/supplements

Our mentoring platform pulls together many strands of my research and clinical work with stem cell technology. Incorporating my success creating stem cell–conditioned media, I began looking at how I could target inflammation, which is the root cause of so many chronic diseases—from arthritis to diabetes to heart disease and some cancers. I knew that if I could tame inflammation and control its effect on the immune response, I would be able to help the tens of millions of people suffering from such diseases and possibly prevent these conditions from developing in the first place.

A Divine Meeting: On a Global Mission to Cultivate Stem Cell Culture

Randy, a successful businessman, had reached out to me after hearing from his friends about my clinical work with stem cells. For years, he'd been trying to manage near-constant discomfort in his knees, where bone-on-bone osteoarthritis had developed. The chronic inflammation had eaten away the cartilage cushioning the bones, causing pain and swelling in both of his knees. He was told that he was at a point where he needed a knee replacement. But Randy wanted to know if there were any other options before he underwent such a risky and painful procedure with its long recovery.

After several consultations, Randy flew from Florida to Beverly Hills to undergo the Stem Cell Lift to his knee at my surgical center.

As I was injecting stem cells into Randy's knees, his wife Wendy chatted with my staff in the front office. Ever curious, Wendy asked about the skincare products that were available. My staff explained that I had created a unique skin serum for wrinkles and skin rejuvenation using stem cell technology that I had developed in our laboratory and research facility.

Wendy was intrigued. And after Randy had completed his procedure, he and Wendy asked me about the skin rejuvenating serum. I then told them the story of how I had discovered the incredible healing properties of stem cells found in adipose tissue and their secretomes for burns and wounds, and how, as a byproduct of our research, I had created the serum for cosmetic use and was hoping to share these powerful and novel products with many more people outside of my practice.

Now even more curious, Randy and Wendy asked if they could try a couple of bottles of the stem cell serum that were designed as a topical cosmetic product.

After Randy's surgical follow-up appointment with me the next day, the couple flew back to Florida with two bottles of serums to try and Randy feeling much better.

A few days later, they called me from Florida.

"This serum is simply amazing," they practically shouted into the phone.

I was delighted to hear this response.

Then Randy continued, "About how many of these bottles do you sell a month?"

"I think about 40," I said.

"How would you like to sell 40,000?" Randy said.

I wasn't sure if he was joking or what he was planning, but I smiled to myself and, not thinking he was serious, I replied, "Sure!"

Sharing the Serum with Millions

I had always wanted to help as many people as possible discover the power of stem cell technology, and Randy and Wendy, successful business owners in their own right, seemed to share my vision. Over the coming days and weeks, I grew to trust this entrepreneurial couple. They seemed inspired to realize my dream of bringing this stem cell technology to the world. And with that in mind, they formed a company to distribute the serum worldwide. Randy, with his vision to advance stem cell science and his early recognition of stem cell technology's rejuvenating potential, named the company Jeunesse, which means "youth" in French, and we called the serum Luminesce (both Jeunesse and Luminesce have since been discontinued).

The power of stem cells lay not only in their ability to become other cells and regenerate but also in the system through which we created the product, including the harvesting method and the creation of a unique environment to direct the stem cells for a specific purpose.

Randy and Wendy also appreciated my use of the term *technology* to capture my method of using stem cells. I knew even then that the power of stem cells lay not only in their ability to become other cells and regenerate but also in the system through which we created the product, including the harvesting method and the creation of a unique environment to direct the stem cells for a specific purpose.

Randy and Wendy's leadership and vision drove Luminesce and Jeunesse to become a worldwide phenomenon, creating hundreds of thousands of ecstatic customers in over 140 countries, whom I was privileged to teach about my stem cell technology and who experienced quick, safe, and lasting results from the expanding line of products I developed.

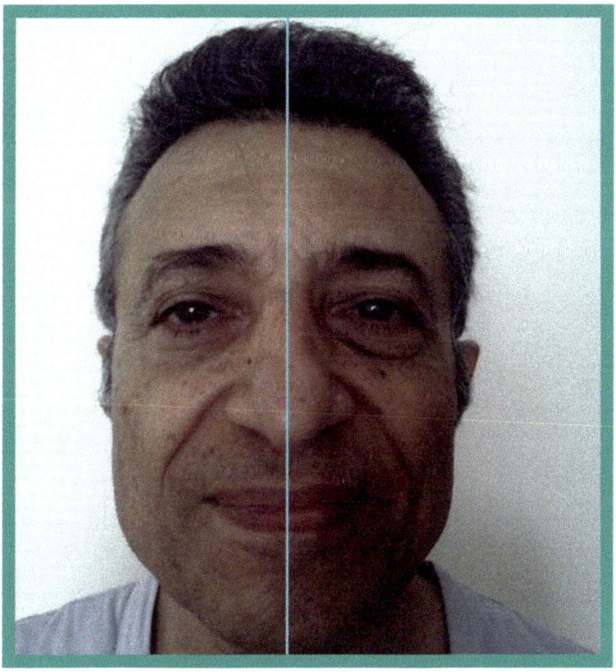

Left: Serum applied for one month. Right: No application

One month after applying my stem cell–based serum to one side of his face, this once-skeptical patient was astonished by the dramatic transformation he experienced.

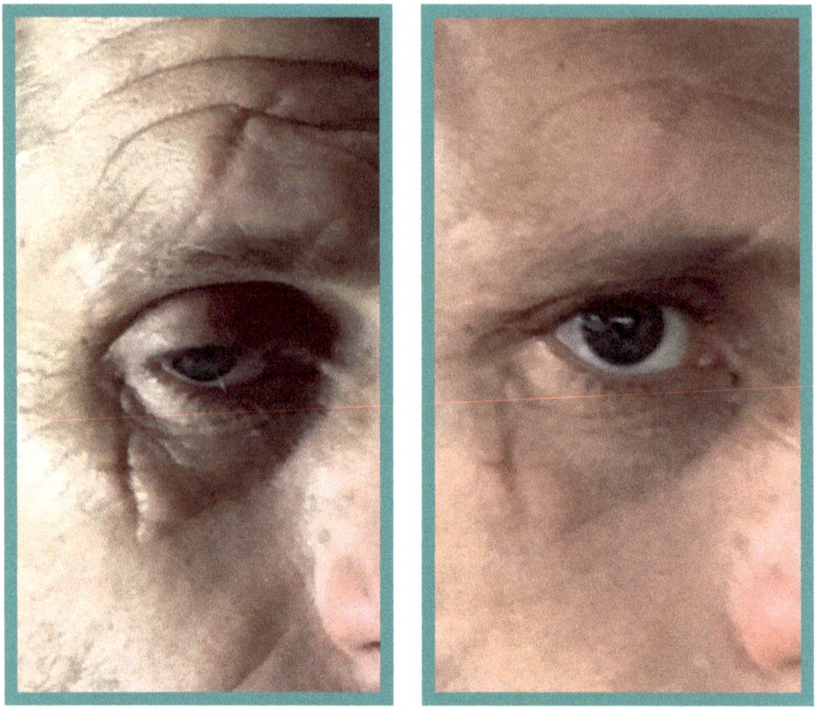

Less than two months after using my stem cell–based serum, this patient shows visible reduction in fine lines and improved skin elasticity and quality.

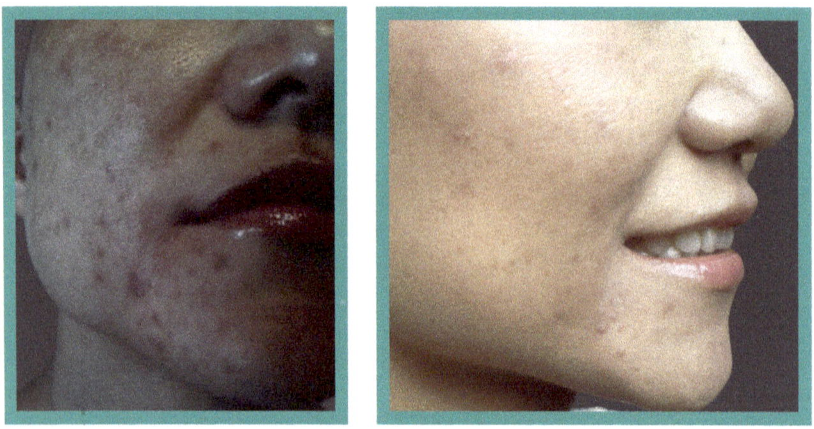

My advanced stem cell–based technology shows remarkable results in restoring both her skin and confidence.

Developing Skin Biotechnology

The success of these early stem cell products motivated my wife Rinat and I to build an even larger, more comprehensive laboratory, where we could continue to conduct stem cell research. We both felt a compelling call to share our know-how with humanity and make stem cell technology better and more accessible. This was very exciting for me, as doing expert-level scientific research in a state-of-the-art lab had always been a dream of mine. Now I could continue to experiment with stem cells and invite other researchers to join me in my efforts. By 2010, we had co-founded our own cosmetics and biotech technology company aimed at developing innovative products and treatments using stem cell language technology. Around that time, we were fortunate to team up with our outstanding CEO, Maya Bodow, who helped us realize our vision. Maya's constant striving for excellence, together with her professionalism and dedication, helped us embark on this new and fascinating journey.

With this I felt my dream of bringing the bounty of stem cell technology to the masses was coming true! As we expanded the global reach for distribution of these early stem cell products, I was invited to speak and present on my research about how stem cell technology was not only an innovative, reliable form of medical treatment but also a source to create innovative products that could help people look and feel better. I was on a global mission to cultivate stem cell culture. For several years, I traveled to Europe, Asia, Australia, and across the Americas. I was eager to see how the hundreds of thousands of people benefiting from my products were doing. I also wanted to gather intelligence, so to speak, about the nuances of their experience. This vast knowledge accumulated from users from all around the world was the most valuable resource to me and the driver for my ongoing mission. Seeing and hearing firsthand from tens of thousands of people of diverse ethnicities and demographics how my evolving stem cell technology had changed their lives for the better inspired me to dig deeper into the science and improve the technology. I'll be forever grateful to Wendy and Randy for believing in me and trusting my technology.

> Seeing and hearing firsthand from tens of thousands of people of diverse ethnicities and demographics how my evolving stem cell technology had changed their lives for the better inspired me to dig deeper into the science and improve the technology.

Pivoting to Plant Stem Cell Technology

As our enterprise and research activities grew, so did the challenges of regulatory hurdles in each country related to the proper use of stem cells. My novel technology and products did not fit into the "check this box" mentality of governmental bureaucracy, and I wanted to find a solution quickly so people around the world could continue to benefit from these stem cell technology–derived products. I asked my team to look at plant stem cell factors. As I dove into the research in my own R&D laboratory, I discovered that plants and humans shared a universal cell language, with human and plant factors having a lot of overlap. This inspired me to reach into the "archives" of medicine and look at how Ayurveda, a 3,000-year-old Eastern medical tradition and approach, incorporates the healing power of plants. I knew, too, that the Ayurvedic tradition also works with the body's natural intelligence and trusts its profound capacity for healing—something I had always believed in. If the body is unwell, it does everything in its power to heal itself; thus, we need to provide it with the right resources and environment to successfully achieve that.

If the body is unwell, it does everything in its power to heal itself; thus, we need to provide it with the right resources and environment to successfully achieve that.

With this intention, it was a natural choice for us to turn to the science of Ayurvedic medicine. We meticulously chose plants known to have beneficial skin effects and started to research. To our amazement, our work showed that all cells—human, animal, plant, or fungus—use one universal language to communicate. They may have different dialects, but using our technology, we can grow any cell or combination of cells and guide them to secrete the instructional factors that when applied to the skin or injected into the tissues, it can direct human cells to carry out the desired tasks. We called these factors *Consortia Factors* because they combine, or *consort*, to form a unique and comprehensive instruction manual to communicate with and direct the cells they come in contact with. Think of each factor as a word and the Consortia Factors as the complete set directions using the combination of these words.

We got right to work in the lab. I wanted to understand more about the dramatic and lasting results that people were experiencing from the serum and continue to explore the world of plant stem cells. It was evident in my clinical practice that patients experienced profound improvement in skin quality, and now I had the power of a state-of-the-art scientific lab to explore why this made sense. After all, as a dermatologist, I knew a lot about how skin loses elasticity and its ability to heal in response to the harsh effects of the environment. Indeed, my interest in sun damage dated back to my undergraduate days, when I first began investigating Parsol 1789 (the date of the French Revolution, as it was the first UVA protecting compound to be tested and later commercialized) for protecting the skin from UVA sun exposure.

Getting It Right: Understanding the Power and Limits of Plants

In the lab, my research team and I began exploring different plants—ashwagandha and tulsi, for example—and experimenting with plant stem cell technology. In keeping with the knowledge that environment matters, we tested different environments and cell-to-cell interactions and combined the stem cells of two or three different plants, not entirely clear on how they would interact with one another. Again, I wanted to understand the various combinations of factors that could enable us to create predictable outcomes. For instance, when co-culturing two different kinds of stem cells that we believed could address inflammation, would we be able to count on the same results, time after time? I always asked the questions, "Will this plant in this condition create this result?"

We tested many different plants, and lo and behold, we discovered that some of them were producing similar effects with each test, showing reproducibility. This line of reasoning reminded me of the connection I had made when I was developing the SCL procedure: it wasn't just the stem cells themselves, but what they were secreting, that was responsible for the changes I was observing in the clinic. So once again, I wanted to know how to use plant stem cells in an analogous manner.

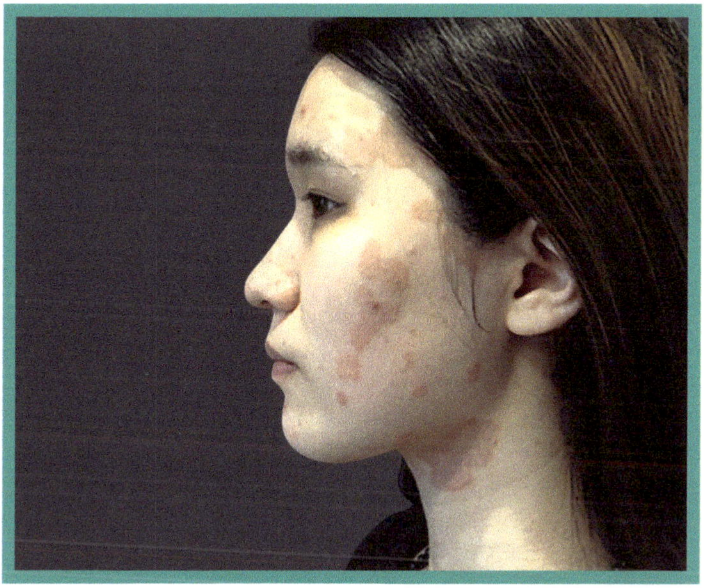

Before

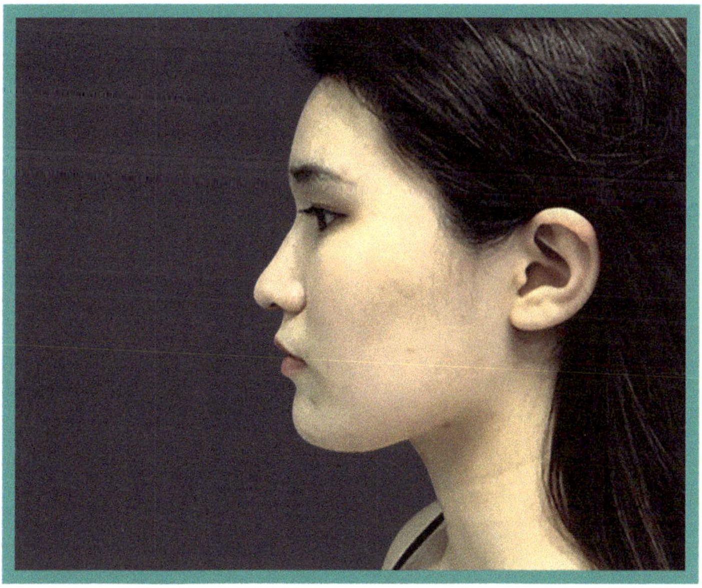

After

Before and after the use of my stem cell–based serum, which not only alleviated the patient's visual symptoms but also treated the pain and itching associated with her sebopsoriasis

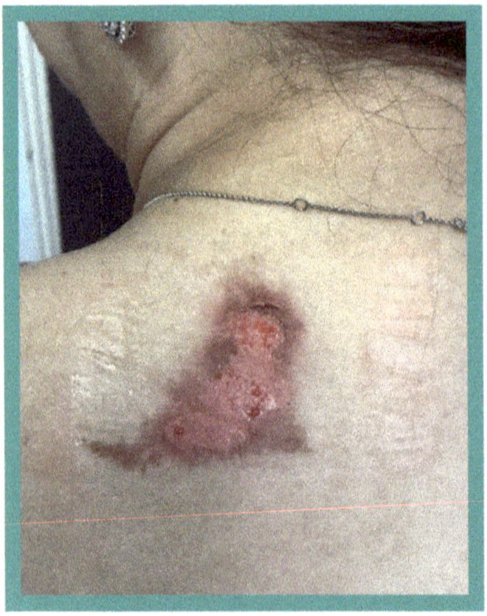

Before

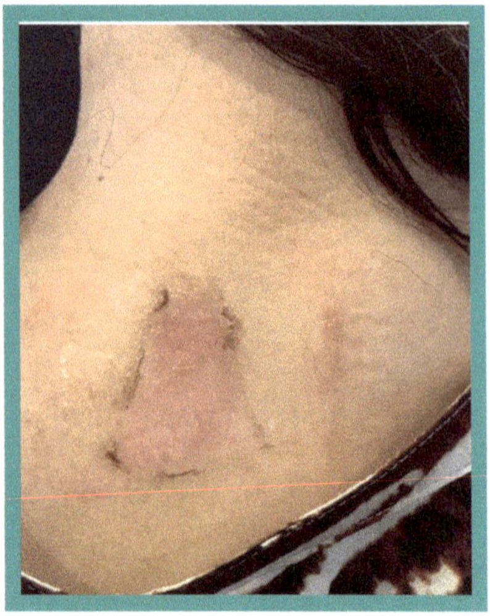

After one week

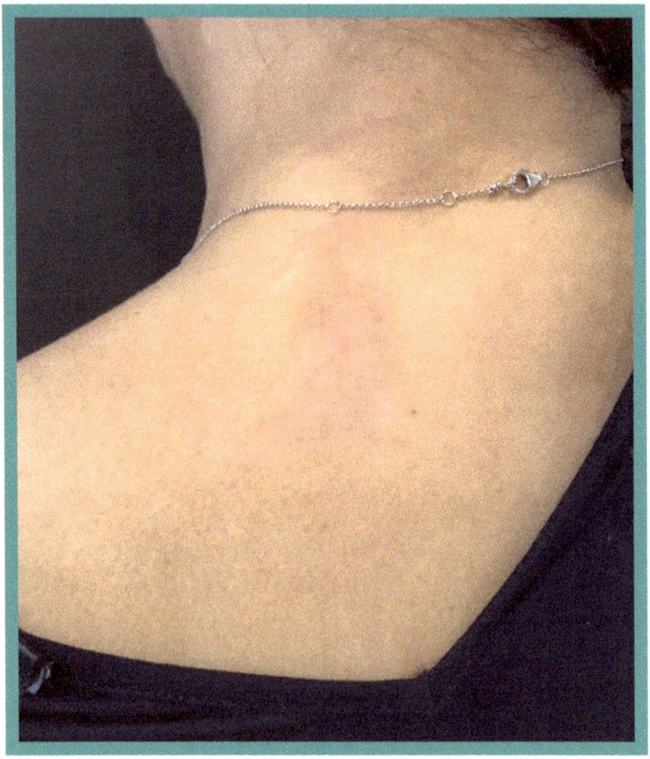

After three weeks

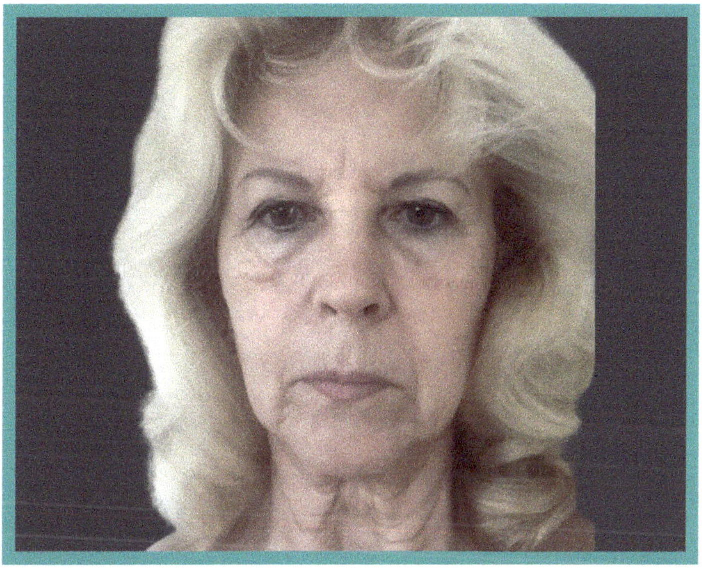

Before

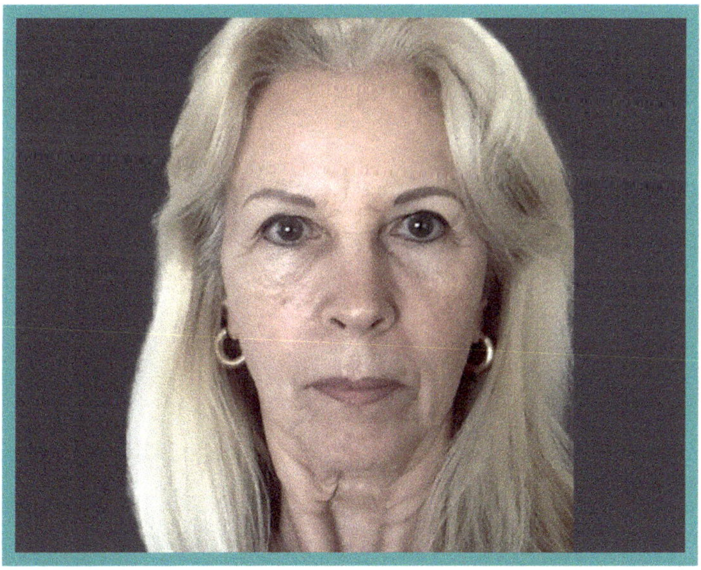

After

Before and after the use of my stem cell–based serum, the transformation is clear. Notice the dramatic reduction in eye bags and the enhanced skin elasticity, thanks to the regenerative and healing power of advanced stem cell technology.

I went back to the effects of the SCL procedure on the skin of my cosmetic patients. I noted that visible improvement in skin texture, quality, and radiance was occurring within days and weeks, not in three to six months as would be expected from any cellular change in the body. This made me realize another incredible fact about Consortia Factors. My holistic approach of neither processing nor adding synthetic compounds to our products was allowing the stem cells to produce the liposomes, exosomes, and other naturally produced carriers for penetrating the skin barrier that were yielding fast and effective results on the skin and hair.

On one of my trips to Australia, I met a woman who showed me this before and after picture of herself after using my skincare products for only six weeks.

She jokingly exclaimed, "This is me," pointing to the after photo, "And this is my mother," pointing to the before picture.

I was impressed but had to be sure it was purely as a result of the products, so I asked her, "This is only from using the products? You did not have any other skin treatments? Botox, fillers, lasers, radiofrequency treatments?"

She smiled and said, "No."

To this day I am amazed by the dramatic skin improvement we see from products created through our research and technology.

Topical Stem Cells for Scar Repair

These stem cell products work well to improve the appearance of scars. This young woman came to see me after she had suffered a severe dog bite. The injury to her face was deep, hard, and disfiguring. Thankfully, I was able to help her heal from these discolored and unsightly scars with a series of nonsurgical treatments in my office. These treatments included Tissue Stimulating Solution (TSS) injections I'd developed, non-ablative laser, and my topical stem cell

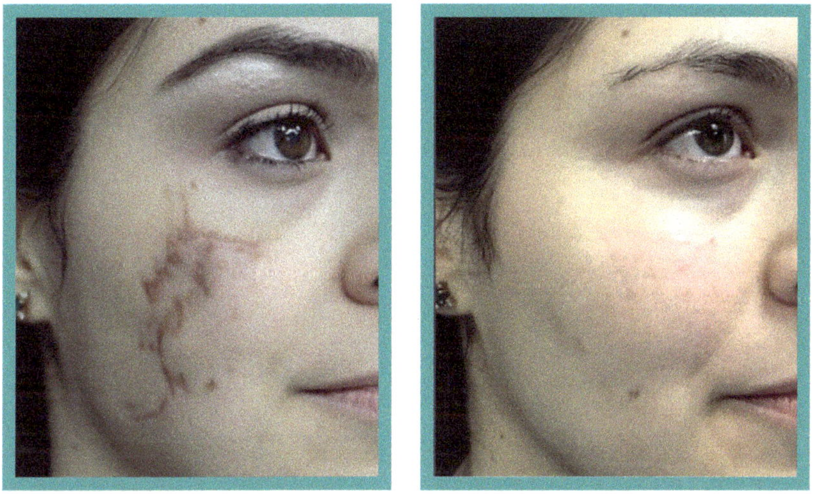

After a traumatic attack left her with visible scarring that both affected her confidence and caused her physical pain, this patient sought alternative treatments. Determined to avoid surgery, she flew to Beverly Hills to see me. Her remarkable results after two years of treatment highlight the transformative power of stem cell technology.

serums. She continued the treatment at home with the topical stem cell serum to repair and restore her skin. Take a look at these before and after photos.

Meet Rosa: Treating Hair Loss

During this time, I was losing my hair despite treatments with topical minoxidil and oral finasteride. I even tried PRP injections, but nothing was working. I decided to research and develop a hair loss product using our stem cell biotechnology. I developed different products and tested them on myself, but nothing seemed to be working and I continued to lose my hair. Around this time, Rosa, my medical assistant, developed alopecia areata, an autoimmune disease that causes patches of hair to fall out. At the time, there were no effective FDA approved drugs for this condition. With conventional treatments using injectable and topical steroids, which stop the immune system from damaging the hair and causing further hair loss to allow the hair to recover, it may take months to see any hair regrowth. Even with such interventions, not all the hair grows back as thick or as dense. Rosa's treatments were not having much effect, and she was still experiencing hair loss. I saw her transform from the confident, bubbly, happy, and positive person she had been to an introverted and depressed shadow of herself. We decided to try the latest version of the hair product that we were developing for my hair loss. After applying the hair serum to her scalp twice a day for one month, we saw that the hair loss stopped and began observing baby hairs emerging.

At two months Rosa showed visible hair growth, and by four months her bald spot had disappeared. We followed her progress, and at one year her hair was thicker and stronger than ever. We were so impressed by Rosa's results that we decided to test the serum on others with androgenic hair loss, also known as natural hormone-induced hair loss. A number of my male and female patients with thinning hair also achieved noticeable improvement and began growing new hair. Confident in these consistent, positive results, we decided to bring this product to the market. It is drug-free, without the potential risks or side effects of the synthetic drugs or hormones available, such as finasteride, the one allowed only for men since it could cause birth defects in women. My hair product, too, saw much success and positive results in the market.

It was clear why the product worked for some and not for others. If the hair was thin, the product thickened and strengthened the follicles; but if the hair had stopped growing completely, a different set of Consortia Factor instructions was needed to stimulate growth. My team and I had figured out the language for thickening existing hair follicles. Now our research aims to find the language that will "wake up" dormant hairs, for the bald men like me, and induce them to grow again. I still want my curls back! :)

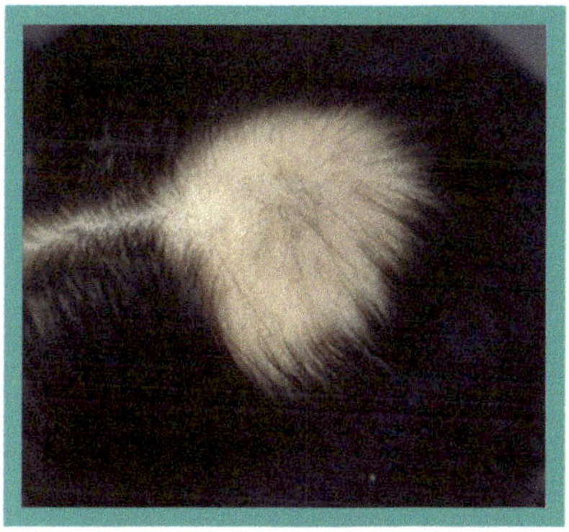

Before

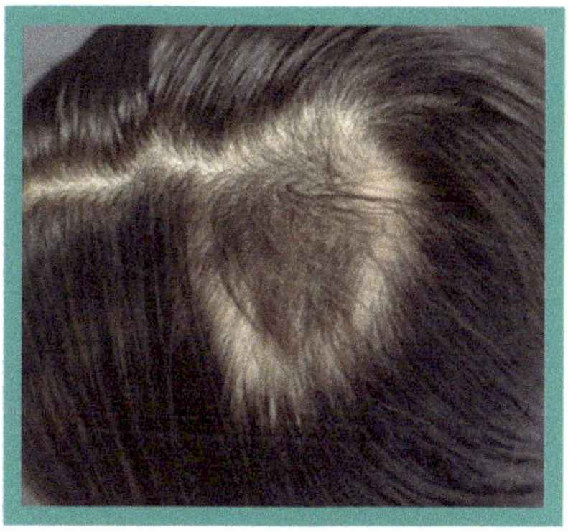

After two months of treatment

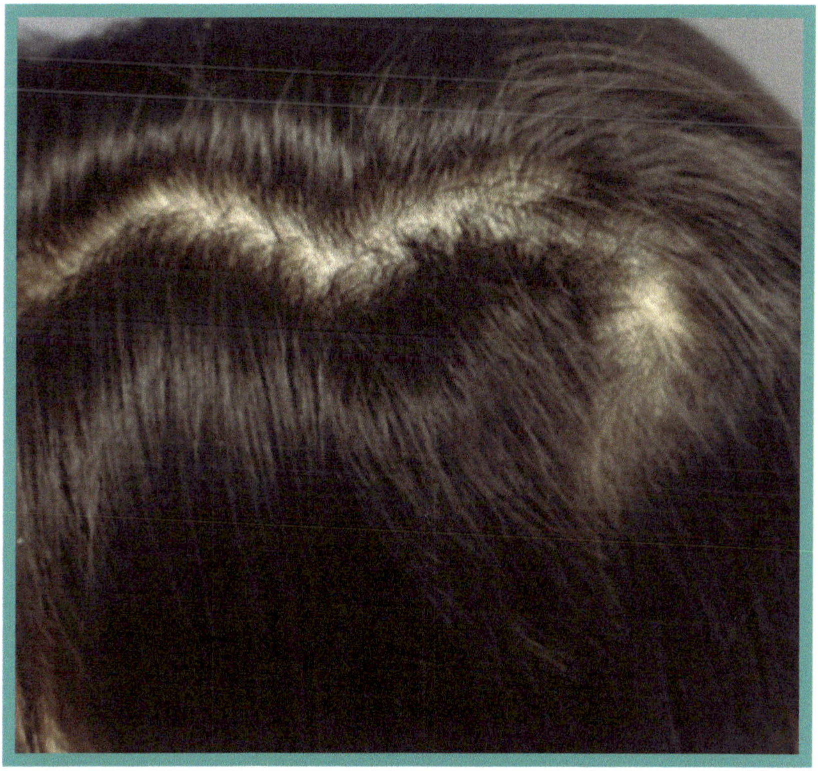

After four months of treatment

Amazing results of using my stem cell–based hair serum to treat the autoimmune disease alopecia areata.

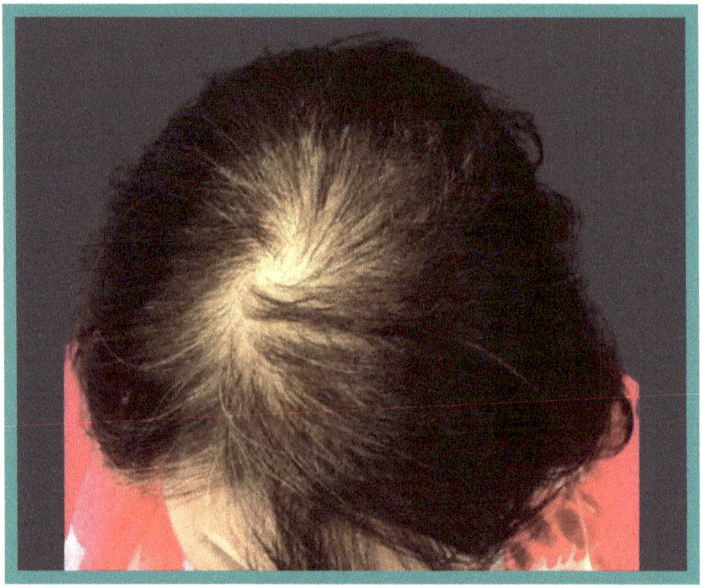

Before

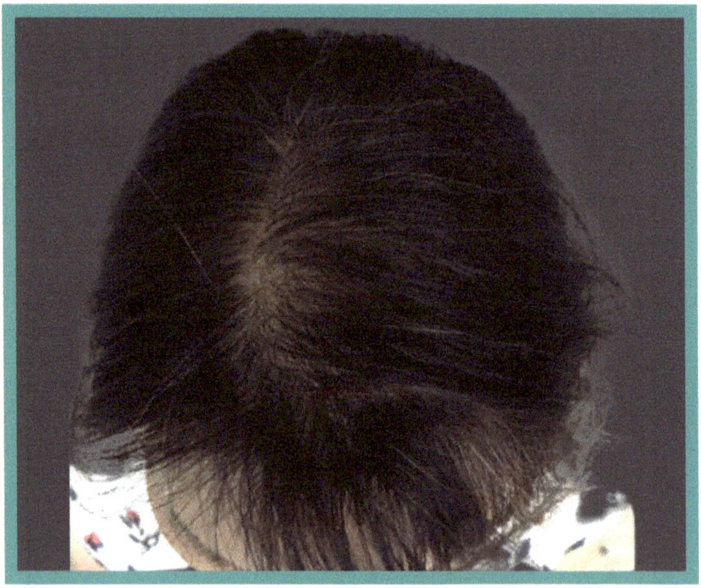

After

Just five months after this patient started to use my stem cell–based hair serum, the improvement in hair thickness and quality is undeniable.

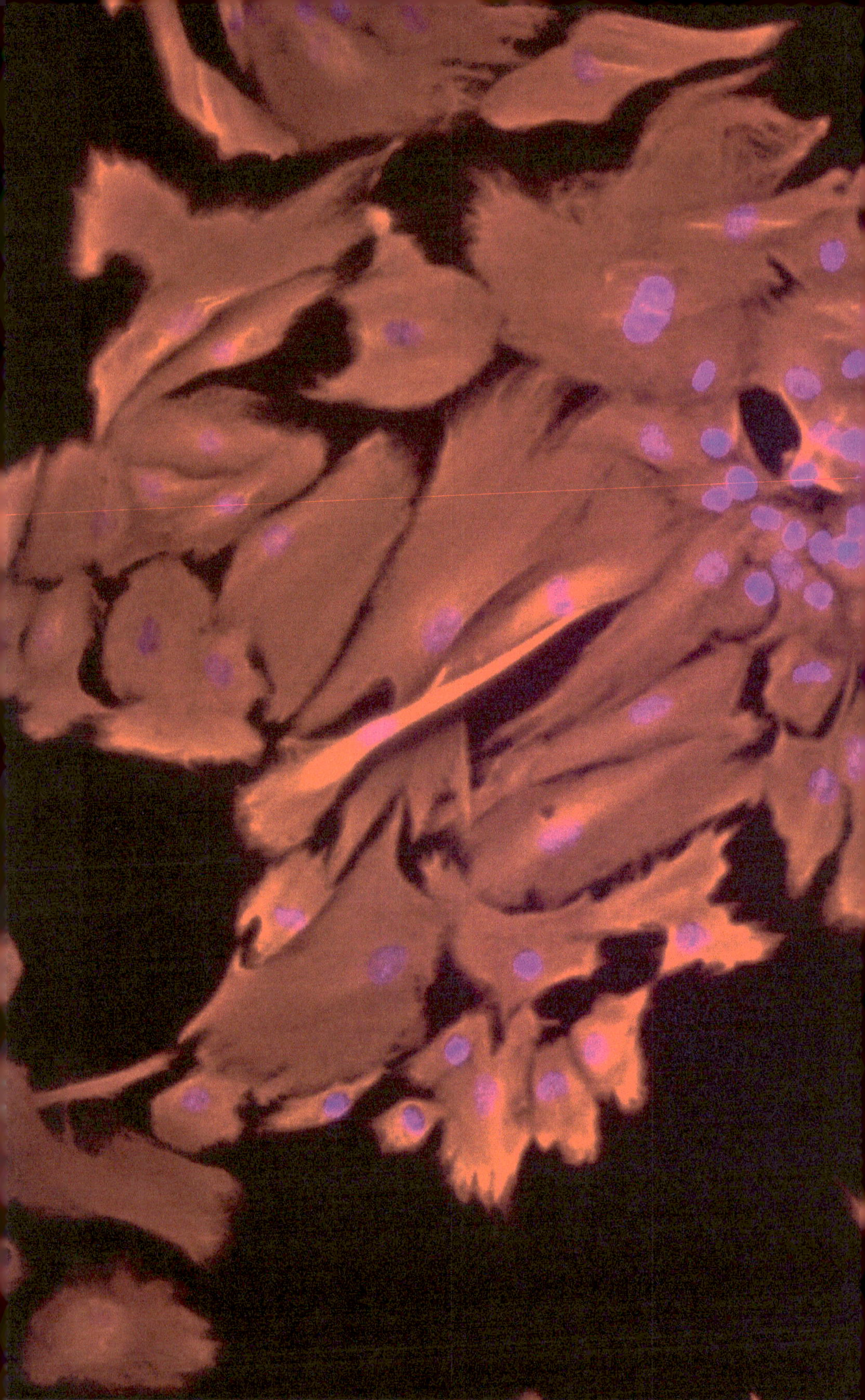

"My mission is to empower people around the world to live their optimum lives and fulfill their dreams. Educating and advocating for yourself is key to keeping healthy, thriving, and enjoying life."

—DR. NATHAN NEWMAN

9

STEM: Science, Technology, Education, and Mentoring

My mission has always been to help as many people as possible benefit from the regenerative potential of stem cell therapy. With our patent, we felt the wind behind our sails to continue to build and broaden that goal. When a colleague in the medical device industry approached me about investing in a new company, I shared the research behind the new patent and its significance for the healthcare sector. It didn't take long for he and I to come up with a plan to create something valuable for physicians and healthcare providers from this patent: a prescriptive line of stem cell agents.

Bringing Our Mission to the World

In 2022, Aesthetics Management Partners (AMP) helped launch this new stem cell technology and medical-grade products to physicians around the world. Since then, Exo|E Technology has become a game changer. Within two years, AMP expanded globally, educating physicians and their patients about our approach to stem cell science and sharing with them the transformative power of stem cells to treat patients and enhance healing.

In the meantime, we continued to engage in other discussions with numerous potential strategic partners to introduce our stem cell therapy to the general public. After years of avoiding the risks and challenges of building a brand that retained our dedication to the integrity of science, we realized that unless we took full control—from start to finish—our technology risked being lost or buried within the bureaucracy of large corporations.

With our small but mighty team—resourceful, dedicated, and immensely talented—we founded The STEM Company and launched our first hero product, STEM ReGenerative Serum in 2023. By the following year, The STEM Company had successfully developed and manufactured a complete line of regenerative skincare products for consumers.

With this step, we were now able to transform our global mission, "STEM for All," into reality. In turn, we were now able to uphold both of our core values: making stem cell technology accessible to everyone and raising awareness of this revolutionary paradigm. With a clear vision, we set out to establish a lasting legacy.

Patenting Our Stem Cell Mentoring Process

My lab was now in a 18,000-square-foot research, development, and manufacturing FDA- and GMP-certified facility next to SpaceX, with a staff of about 10 researchers. With my vision of utilizing stem cell language to create off-the-shelf products for the benefit of the masses, we developed a platform technology to grow stem cells and direct them to produce a specific set of signals we could bottle and apply to the tissues to induce the desired response. We also had to overcome many challenges of using live cell cultures. In particular, it was important to create an environment where the cells could grow in a clean medium, free of unwanted chemicals and animal products. We also needed to figure out how to make a reproducible, consistent, and effective product and confirm that the product remained active, stable, safe, and effective over time. It was also important that this enriching product be unadulterated, natural, and not processed. In order to achieve all of these goals, we had to control the entire process from the cell to the bottle.

After much research and testing, we had succeeded in creating a one-of-a-kind platform and process in which we can start from any cell we choose; mentor them in cell culture to produce the unique CFx language in a consistent, predictable, reproducible, and scalable manner; and bottle this novel regenerative product for the benefit of the consumer. This is a first in the industry, and as noted earlier, we were granted a patent for our unique and novel technology.

STEM for All

With The STEM Company, we were now able to bring all of my knowledge of, experience with, and vision for regenerative medicine and biotechnology to all of humanity. Just as I used my gift of observation to go from the clinic to the lab, I was now able to go from the lab to the clinic and then to the public to complete my global mission of cultivating stem cell culture. For this reason, we called the new skincare brand STEM, which stands for:

- Science
- Technology
- Education
- Mentoring

Using the ReGenerative Serum, the STEM Natural Intelligence hero product

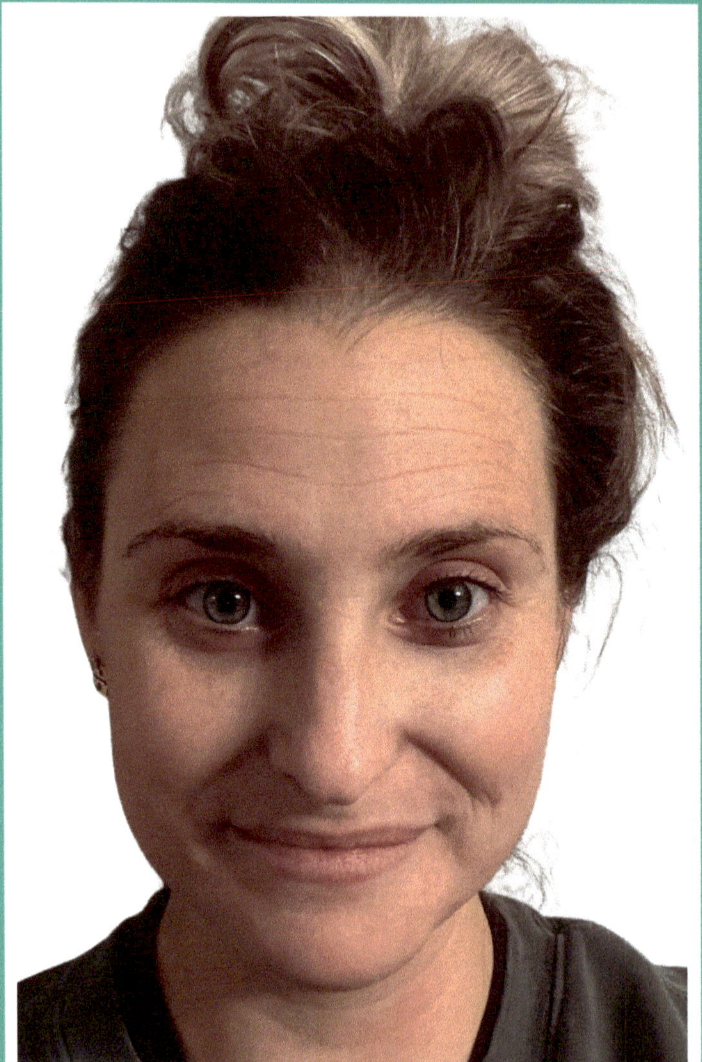

Before

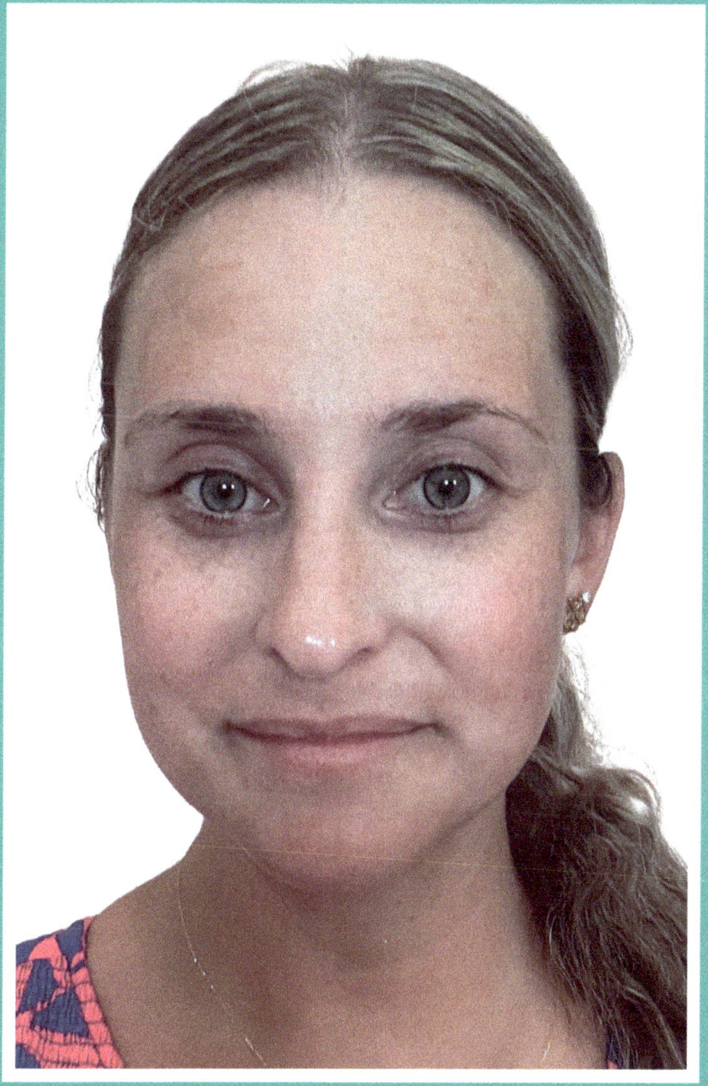

After one month

Noticeable rejuvenation of skin and facial appearance

Using the ReGenerative Serum, the STEM Natural Intelligence hero product

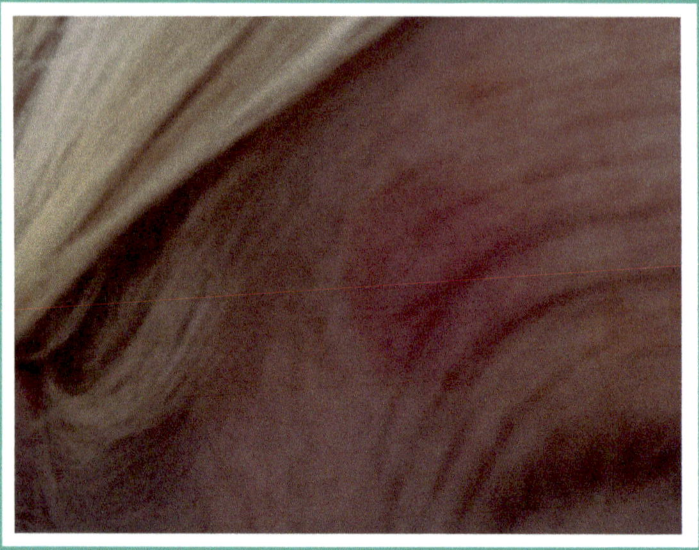

Before

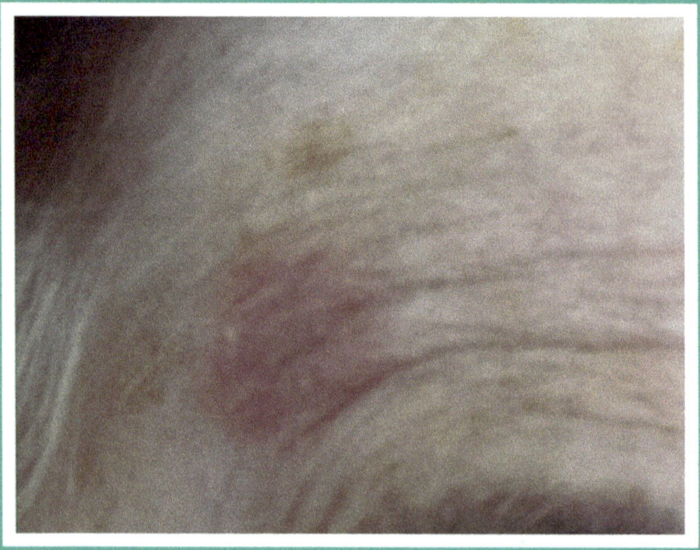

After two weeks

After one month

Reduced signs of burns and scarring appearance

Using the ReGenerative Serum, the STEM Natural Intelligence hero product

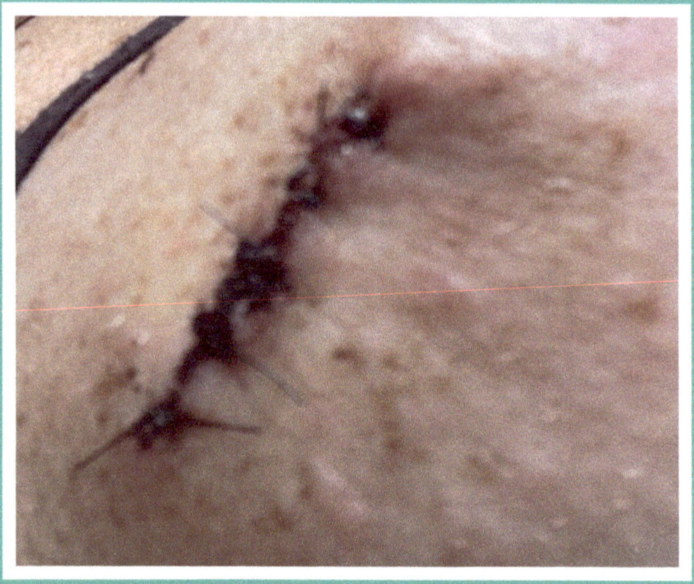

Before

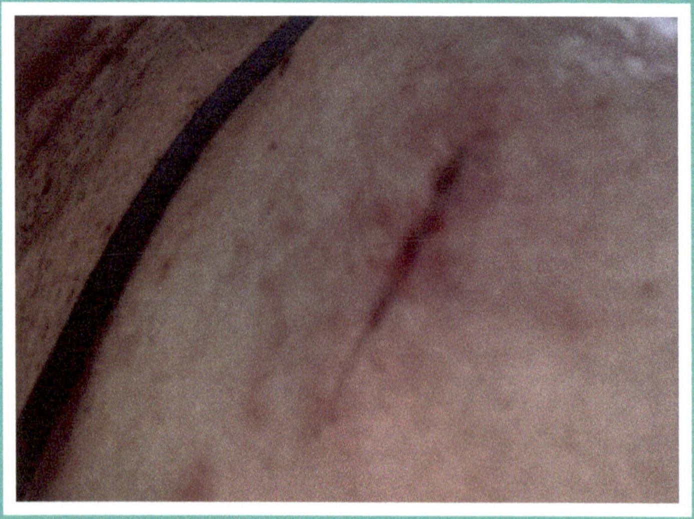

After two weeks

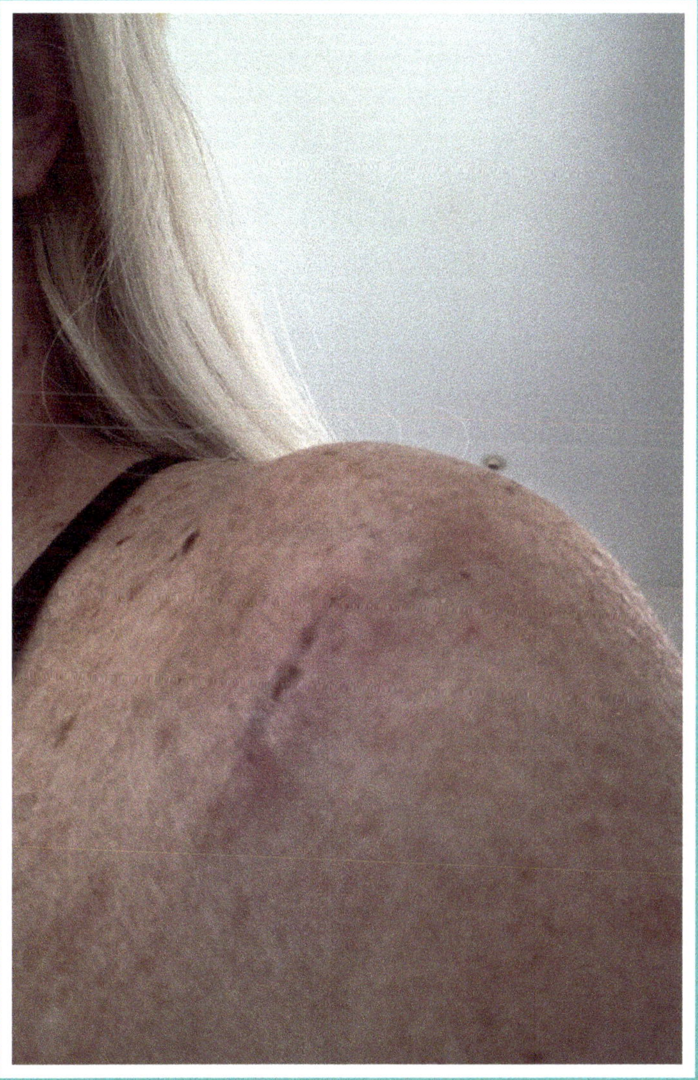

After one month

Improving and expediting healing of skin appearance post-surgery

STEM is the culmination of my three decades of medical study, scientific research and development, and regenerative medicine practice. Powered by the natural intelligence of regenerative stem cell factors, STEM represents the evolution of modern-day personal care, health, vitality, and longevity from an anti-aging approach to one that is regenerative, becoming a trailblazer in beauty and wellness. Whereas anti-aging skincare relies on harsh chemicals and acids to "talk at" your skin and body in order to fight signs of aging, our regenerative skincare products utilize the cell's own language to "work with" your body to balance, nourish, renew, restore and rejuvenate—without any harsh chemicals. It is plant based, cruelty free, clean, safe and family and pet friendly.

Whereas anti-aging skincare relies on harsh chemicals and acids to "talk at" your skin and body in order to fight signs of aging, our regenerative skincare products utilize the cell's own language to "work with" your body to balance, nourish, renew, restore and rejuvenate—without any harsh chemicals.

Another part of my mission is to educate and help people develop tools to be healthy and live optimally. During my years of treating patients in my clinic, it has become painfully clear that women's health is not well understood, studied, described, addressed, or taught, especially for perimenopausal and menopausal women. Just like the paracrine effects of stem cell factors are vital for cellular balance, function, and health, so are the endocrine effects of hormones, especially in the flux of perimenopause. And in the endeavor to educate the public and mentor clinicians, I will dedicate a portion of the profits of our company for research, education, mentoring, and grants to help improve women's health and optimize the quality of their lives.

Biopharmaceutical Medications

In addition to these personal care products, we are also developing and testing medical treatments that will go through biological drug pathways for FDA approval. We are committed to the safety and efficacy of all of our products—whether they are over the counter, cosmetic, or medicinal and prescribed by doctors. Currently, we are developing therapies that use our stem cell mentoring technology to

- Treat burns
- Improve breathing
- Heal wounds
- Repair muscle
- Heal bone
- Restore bone for dentistry
- Heal cartilage

Some of these medicines are topical, while others are injectables or inhalers. As with my other uses of stem cells, the cell-free Consortia Factors containing the cellular language for treatments that we are testing are uniquely developed through our patented stem cell mentoring process to target specific disease conditions. Again, my goal in creating a range of products is to widen access so more and more people suffering from disease, injury, or the negative effects of aging can benefit from this revolutionary technology.

Consortia Factors to Treat Wounds and Burns

The scientific study of stem cell therapy used for tissue repair and wound healing has grown significantly in the last few decades. We have continued to make progress in identifying the numerous and nuanced ways in which stem cells can be utilized to achieve full restoration of structures and their function.

Most wounds address damage to the soft tissue of the skin, which forms about 15 percent of the total body mass (weight) and covers the entire surface area of the body. And although the skin has great self-repairing and self-renewing capacity, damage due to burns and lacerations that penetrate past the skin surface can cause debilitating scars that traditional medicine has had limited success treating.

To put this into perspective, it is estimated that more than $1.5 billion is spent annually in the US to treat burn injuries, including second-degree burns, and the average cost of $24,000 for the burn victim's hospital stay is twice that of other causes. One out of four burn victims in the United States are children under 18 years of age, and the worldwide mortality rate is seven times higher for children in lower to middle-income countries.

Table 2: Characteristics of burns by degree

	1ST DEGREE	2ND DEGREE	3RD DEGREE
Burn depth	Epidermis	Dermis	Hypodermis
Clinical appearance	Erythematous No blister	Erythematous Blisters (wet)	White or black No blister
Sensation	Mild pain	Extreme pain	No sensation
Intervention	Topical skin care	May need surgery	Needs surgery
Average healing time	Two weeks	Six weeks	Will not heal without intervention
Scar formation	No scar	Scar	Scar
Hospitalization	None	>15% TBSA	All

Burns and wounds affecting the surface of the skin (or epidermal layer) are typically capable of regeneration without scarring, but deeper dermal injuries heal by scar formation. Complications associated with deep skin burns and those affecting larger surface areas of the body include infection, hypovolemia (low blood pressure and blood flow from dehydration), hypothermia and electrolyte imbalance from loss of skin barrier to the environment, and breathing difficulties. These wounds usually heal with scar formation that may cause physical and emotional stress and disabilities, such as restricted movement of an extremity from contracture scars. The last medication to treat burns to be approved by the FDA was silver sulfadiazine (commercial name Silvadene) in 1973, and only a handful of devices have been approved for burn treatment.

In my clinic, I observed the successful and robust wound healing that I was able to achieve with the patient's own stem cells. However, I knew that most of the healing was carried out via the innate regenerative capacity of stem cell secretory factors. In my early years, I successfully treated non-healing ulcers merely by placing stem cells on top of the wound. It's for this reason that I set out to create an off-the-shelf medication using stem cell healing language that would bring skin burn and wound healing treatment into the 21st century. This regenerative product provides a number of advantages, offering the potential to impact the health and lives of millions of people worldwide. Think of how many people suffering from burn wounds could be helped using a serum they can get over the counter!

As I was developing and testing this product, I came across some patients who used our product with fantastic results, which gave me the passion, zeal, and determination to bring this amazing technology to the world. The photos below show a three-year-old boy who had a hot liquid second-degree burn, resulting in blisters and skin loss to his torso, arm, and forearm. His family are patients who were aware of my work with stem cells and brought him to me for treatment. He was in a lot of pain and discomfort. I provided them with our topical serum to apply on the wounds, and within a couple of days his pain and discomfort had subsided. The skin healed rapidly and without scarring.

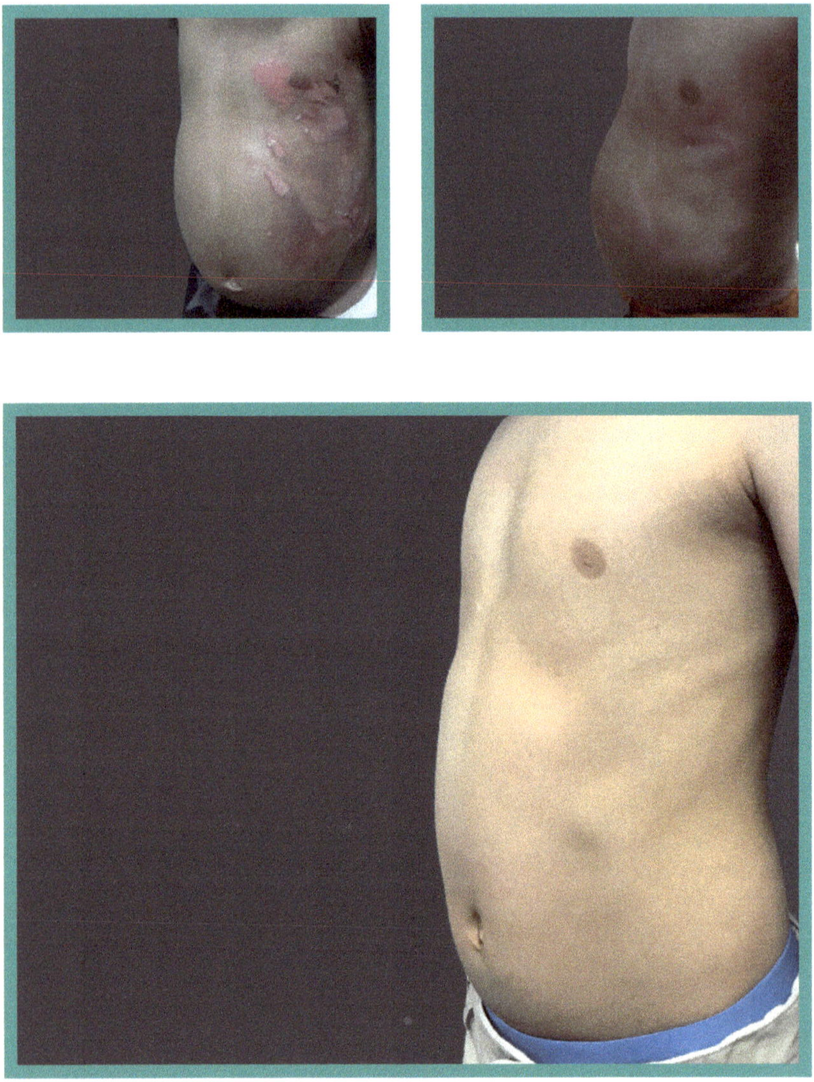

Despite the potential for lifelong scarring, my stem cell–based serum not only alleviated the pain from this 1-year old's burn, but also five years later, has left no visible evidence of the injury.

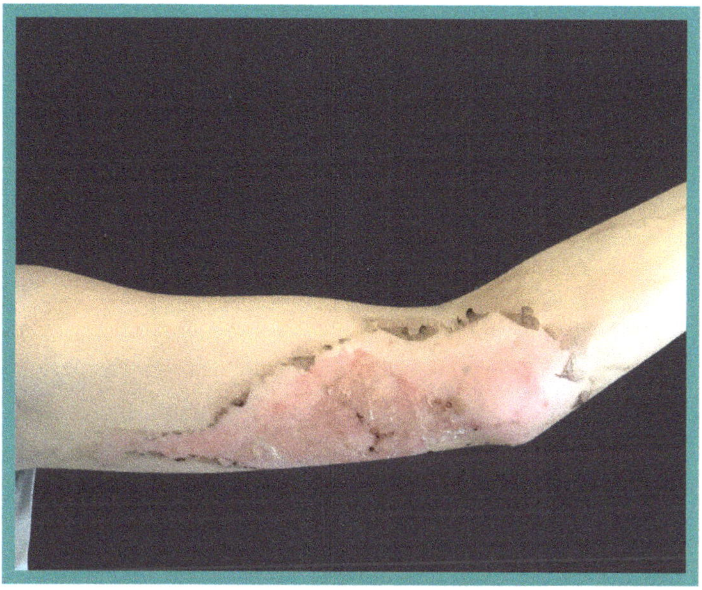

Before

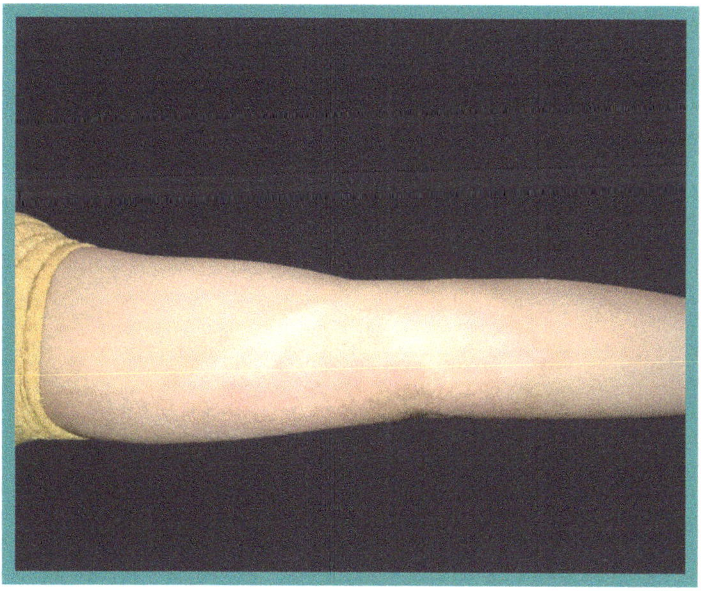

After

Three weeks after an accidental spill resulting in a second-degree burn, the patient's skin demonstrates accelerated healing, attributed to my advanced stem cell–based technology.

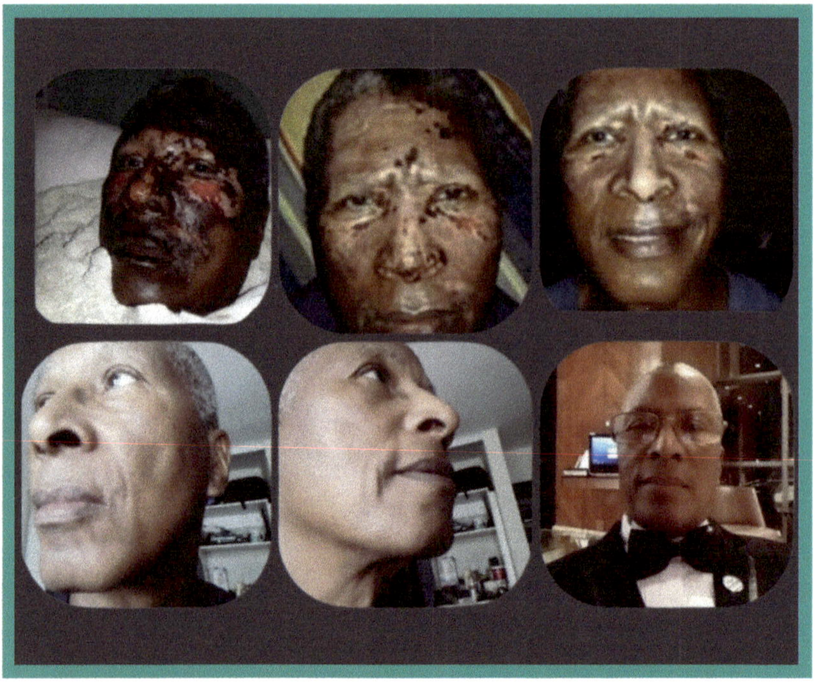

Just 1.5 months after suffering excruciating second-degree burns from a pyrotechnic incident, this patient shows no visible signs of damage.

While I was traveling to Panama to give a talk about my stem cell research and products, one of the attendants, dressed in a tuxedo, approached me at a dinner and showed me his pictures. He had suffered burns to his face and neck during a pyrotechnic accident with fireworks. He was hospitalized in the intensive care unit for nine days and then transferred to the ward. He told me he'd felt that at this point the only thing that might help save his face from scarring was to use my product, so he had. I could not believe my eyes. He had no scars, no skin discoloration, no sign of damage to his skin.

I have also seen my stem cell serums heal burns caused by radiation during breast cancer treatment. In this case, the patient had a total mastectomy (surgical removal of all breast tissue) and then radiation to the breast area to treat the cancer. Radiation burns are very painful and usually result in long-term skin discoloration, scarring, and sensitivity. When she used our product, the pain, burning, and sensitivity resolved in a few days, and within two weeks the skin burn was resolved.

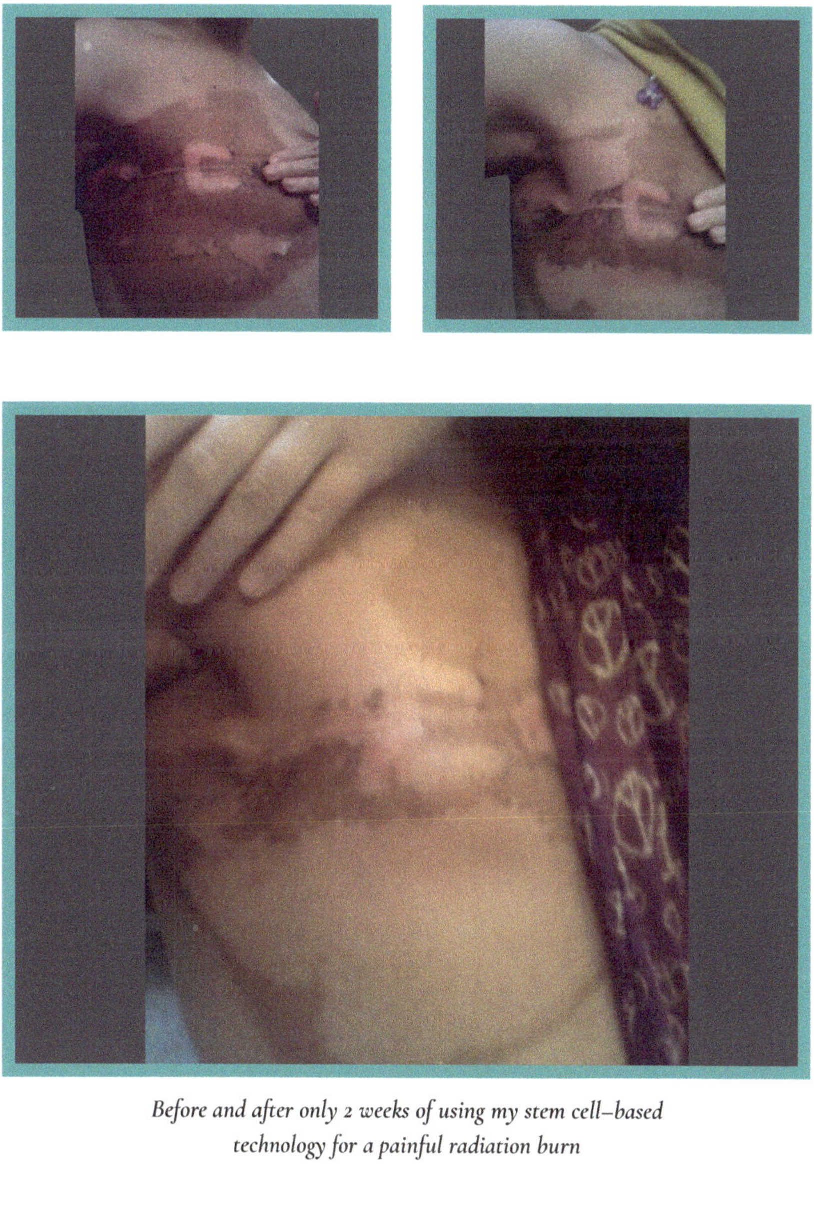

Before and after only 2 weeks of using my stem cell–based technology for a painful radiation burn

Without this novel stem cell technology, these patients would suffer for weeks and would take months to heal. They would have long-term skin damage that would have a lifelong negative psychosocial impact, such as being self-conscious about the scars or losing self-confidence, preventing them from living optimally.

As I write this book, we are going through the FDA approval process to make this transformative remedy for burn and wound repair available to all.

Functional Foods for Health and Balance

We know that plants are a rich source of nutrients that are essential for human life. We also know that plants contain powerful bioactive phytochemicals that help prevent disease and enhance treatment once disease has taken hold. Since plants are exposed to continual environmental changes, they become inherently protective and therapeutic. Obviously, many ancient cultures have been using plants as medicine with astonishing results. For centuries, plants have been used in India, China, and Peru, for example, to treat parasites, malaria, and other ailments. What's in plants that's so potent they can cure and heal disease? The short answer is this: phytochemicals. These naturally occurring substances have been shown through research to regulate stem cell signaling, metabolism, and cells' ability to communicate with one another. These capacities have been shown to promote stem cell growth, differentiation, and reprogramming—all of which are how stem cells stay regulated and naturally work to protect and support the immune system.

Phytochemicals, also referred to as natural compounds, can be categorized in four groups, according to their biochemical structures:

- **Phenolic acids or polyphenols.** These powerful antioxidants help protect against oxidative stress, which can lead to inflammation; they can be found in fruit skins, seeds, and the leaves of green vegetables.

- **Flavonoids.** There are over 5,000 types of these compounds that carry out important functions in plants, such as combating environmental stress, attracting pollinators, and regulating cell growth. Foods that are high in flavonoids include apples, berries, soybeans, citrus fruits, leafy green vegetables, and onions.
- **Alkaloids.** Made up of amino acids (the building blocks of proteins), these compounds may sound familiar: l-lysine and l-tyrosine.
- **Carotenoids.** These naturally occurring pigments act as both antioxidants and anti-inflammatory agents. Known for their bright colors—yellow, orange, red, and purple—they can be found in carrots, pumpkins, tomatoes, and red paprika, to name a few sources.

The functional food supplements that I am creating with my research partners are designed to combine and concentrate these compounds to be highly effective.

Bringing Stem Cells to Animals

All of us, especially our CEO Maya, love our pets, so we are also very motivated to develop a line of stem cell–based products that can help animals heal from injuries and lessen their pain (from arthritis, for instance). Given our love for animals, we want to offer all of them a better quality of life as they age. The fact that our products are plant based and clean makes them very safe and pet friendly.

The Future Is Ours

Throughout history, major scientific breakthroughs have propelled medicine forward and saved many lives. Antibiotics, anesthesia, pharmaceutical medications, lasers, and endoscopic surgery have all had major transformative benefits for humankind, and now robotics and regenerative medicine are ushering in a new era of longevity and vitality we will all benefit from. Scientific advancements are enabling the transition from reactive treatments that simply alleviate symptoms to proactive treatments that address the cause of many ailments.

Much as I transitioned from a two-dimensional approach of cutting and pulling to a three-dimensional approach of restoring and rejuvenating with the Stem Cell Lift, so too will our Consortia Factors transform medical and surgical approaches to healing and health.

Much as I transitioned from a two-dimensional approach of cutting and pulling to a three-dimensional approach of restoring and rejuvenating with the SCL, so too will our Consortia Factors transform medical and surgical approaches to healing and health.

As we've discussed, these technologies already exist and as soon as the regulatory and medical worlds become more aware and adopt them, they will be available to all. You can benefit from off-the-shelf products that—unlike synthetic pharmaceuticals that talk *at* your body to address only one component of the problem and have undesired side effects and complications—talk *with* your body, using the language of your cells in a complete and balanced manner, to heal you with minimal risk or side effects.

In addition to the cosmetics formulated from plant stem cells and using Consortia Factor technology, my team and I have already created products that treat many serious health conditions (including burns, wounds, lung issues, joint problems such as meniscus tears, muscle tears, bone issues, teeth and gum problems, neurological conditions, and eye ailments); rejuvenate skin; restore hair; promote gut health; and support pet health. Our Exo|E technology—which, as I mentioned, is a prescription-based line developed for doctors and other healthcare providers—offers patients more specialized stem cell therapies.

Stem cell therapy and Consortia Factors technology will directly affect and advance the science of epigenetics, mitochondrial function, apoptosis and cellular programming, cellular senescence, and senolytics, as the cellular language is what modulates these functions in your body. The language of the cell is created through genes and epigenetic translation. Consortia Factors may induce a desired cellular dialogue that will positively influence these functions to improve your health. Stem cell technology coupled with gene therapy will change medicine, health, and longevity just as the mobile phone changed communication.

Using stem cell technology, we will be able to treat problems of immune dysregulation, leaky gut, neurodegenerative decline, and physical wear and tear in a new manner that will result in longevity with vitality. The more you do to maintain your health, the longer you will live to benefit from this revolution.

Since we were issued the patent for our stem cell mentoring technology, my research team and I have been busy imagining all the ways it can be applied to maintaining good health and to regenerating and healing the body. We are offering as many people as possible new ways to think about disease and aging. With those goals in mind, we have already created different categories of products that offer solutions to common but stubborn problems as well as innovative approaches to serious diseases, including cancer and neurological disorders. In my humble opinion, the potential of stem cell therapy is limitless!

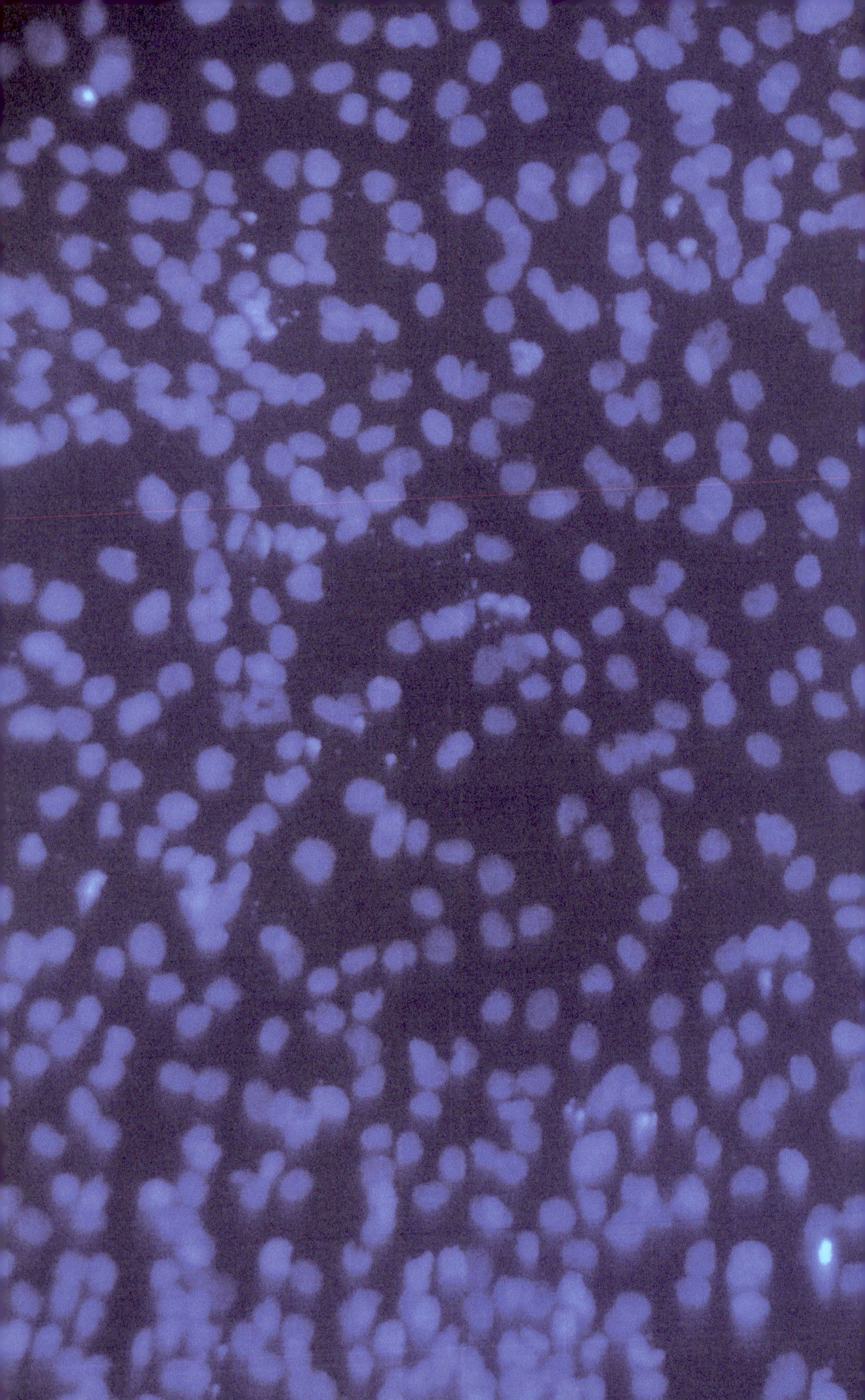

"Stem cell natural intelligence is a new paradigm in regenerative medicine. It aims to cultivate independent research and inspire innovative thinking by raising awareness."

—DR. NATHAN NEWMAN

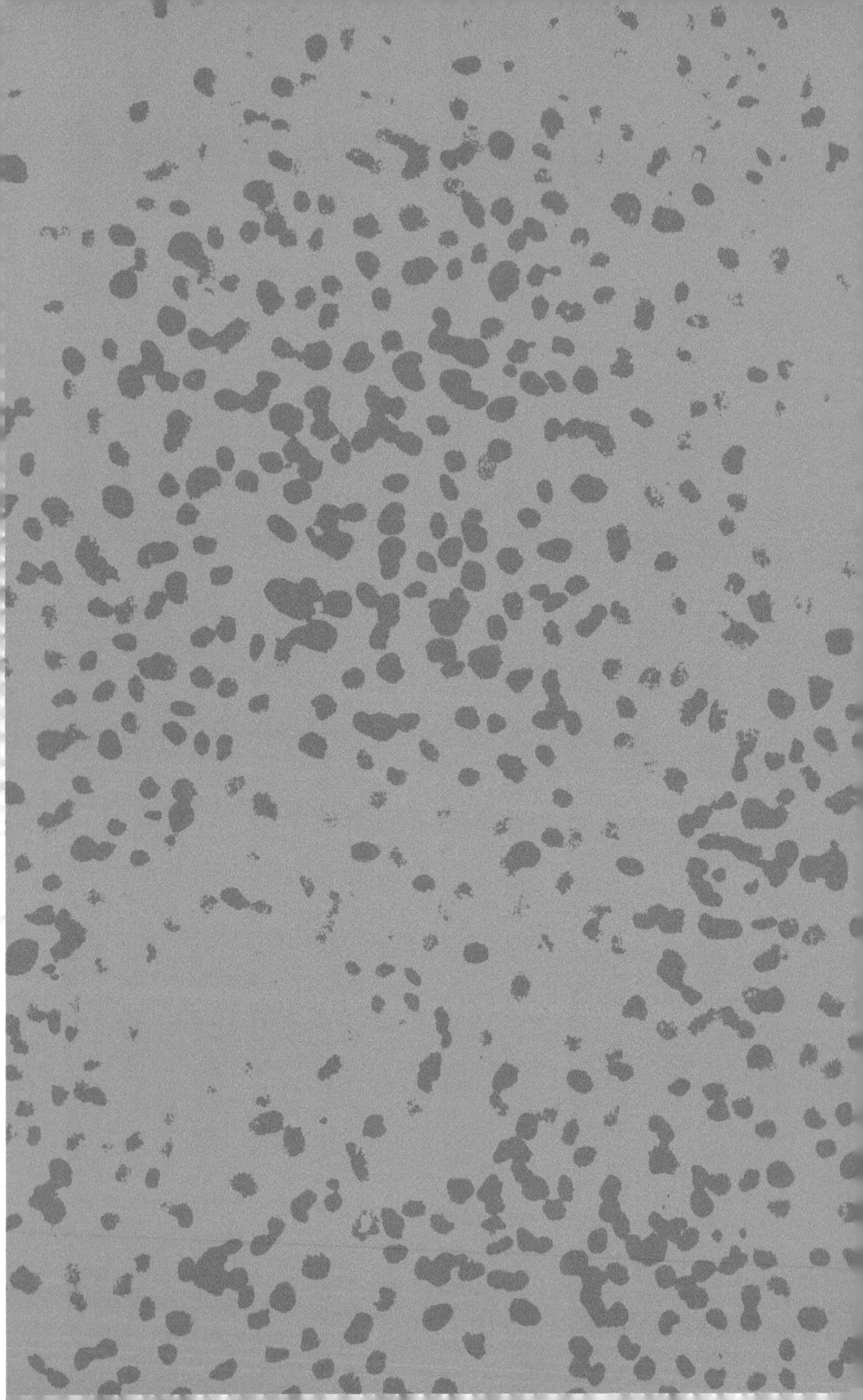

10

How Your Lifestyle Can Synergize Stem Cell Health

When my patients ask me for advice on how to enhance their stem cell therapy, I always begin by reminding them that feeling and looking their best begins with balancing and honoring their body. Every one of us can benefit from stem cell technology—whether you are concerned about a health issue, want to offset aging, or wish to achieve a better quality of life. Of course, stem cell therapy will enable you to heal faster and look better, and it may even help you live a long and vibrant life. But when you also maintain a healthy lifestyle—optimizing nutrition, exercise, and sleep—you amplify the quality of your stem cells and the effects of stem cell therapy.

It's All About Balancing Nutrition, Exercise, and Sleep

As soon as a patient sits down with me to learn more about stem cell therapy, I make sure to touch upon the importance of a healthy lifestyle to support any procedure or product. Why? Because the Stem Cell Lift procedure and other uses of plant and human stem cell therapy are always enhanced through how we eat, how active we are on a regular basis, and how well we sleep. What we put in our bodies and how we treat them makes all the difference in how we age, prevent disease, and heal. I must admit that I'm not perfect—far from it! But I do strive to eat whole, clean foods most of the time and stay away from processed, packaged foods as much as possible. And even though I am very busy—working in my clinic, traveling to international medical conferences, and spending time with my family—I try to work out regularly. The importance of exercise cannot be underestimated! And sleep? That's the time when your body resets and recalibrates, and the older we get, the more our brains and bodies rely on this restorative period to come back into balance. Sleep is key to cellular resilience.

> When you also maintain a healthy lifestyle—optimizing nutrition, exercise, and sleep—you amplify the quality of your stem cells and the effects of stem cell therapy.

Think about your lifestyle choices as opportunities to restore balance to your overall brain–body system. Remember the concept of homeostasis, and how the human body is driven to maintain it? Being in balance is inextricably linked to the body's ability to achieve and maintain homeostasis. And the better you eat, sleep, and exercise, the better able you are to stay in homeostasis. Your body works best when you are physically active; indeed, we are all meant to move.

I believe in doing everything in moderation to be able to make that our lifestyle. Exercise is great, but people often overlook simple changes that can make a difference: walking just 30 minutes a day or taking the stairs on a regular basis instead of the elevator can help your cellular health.

I like to keep things simple. I am not a fan of extreme diet or exercise routines. Instead, I believe that people are more likely to begin and stick to a healthy regimen if the advice makes sense and feels more or less easy. So, I am not suggesting you make radical changes; rather, I think it's best to take some time to consider the idea of balance and moderation and all that it can do for you, once you embrace it.

Pay Attention to Your Body

I always speak to my patients about developing a healthy relationship with their body, which starts by accepting your body the way it is right now. And although it's important to your overall health to maintain a healthy weight for your body type, again think about what you can and cannot change about your body. You may remember from high school biology the three general body types—ectomorph, mesomorph, and endomorph—fancy ways to say that some of us are naturally small-boned, others have a medium frame, and still others have a larger or broader physique. Being fit and healthy does not require changing your innate physique but rather accepting your shape and working with it so that you feel good in your body. I live in the heart of Los Angeles, a city where women and men of all ages can get distracted by, or even obsessed with, manipulating their bodies to try to reach an ideal that can undermine their health, never mind their confidence and self-esteem. I spend time with my patients talking about nurturing a healthy attitude toward food—and their bodies.

It's also crucial that you pay attention to what your body is telling you: Do certain foods make you bloated or gassy? Do other foods cause skin breakouts? Your body will tell you when something you ingest is not good for you, so get in the habit of paying attention to how certain foods make you feel. There are nuances to how your body reacts to different foods and even the timing of when you eat.

Again, moderation is key. Be flexible so you can give yourself room to have treats on holidays or celebrations; eating and exercising well is not all or nothing. Be forgiving of yourself: If you're tired one week because of work deadlines, for example, allow yourself to rest and relax. Given my heavy travel schedule, it would be easy for me to be hard on myself for not sticking to my typical clean diet and regular exercise regimen. But I've learned that going easy on myself and thinking about these breaks in routine actually makes me more aware of what my body needs.

For patients who are concerned about their weight, I keep things simple. I don't recommend dieting, but I do help my patients get in touch with their satiety signal. By satiety, I mean the internal signal your brain sends your body to tell you you're full or satisfied after a meal. It's common for people to eat past their satiety point, which can lead to overeating and weight gain. When we eat fast, barely chewing our food, we can also dull our sense of fullness, which in turn will make us eat more than we really intend. Eating slowly will help your mind–gut connection communicate that your stomach is stretched full of food and that you are no longer hungry. This usually takes about 20 minutes, so if you eat fast, you tend to overeat because your stomach hasn't yet sent the satiety signal. Take your time and eat in a mindful way.

In today's culture, with so much focus on staying youthful and being thin, it can be difficult to resist being fat phobic. Body dysmorphia—a condition that affects the way you perceive and think about your body—is real, and it's exacerbated by social media and the new weight loss wonder drugs. People who suffer from body dysmorphia can't stop thinking about the way they look or how they compare to others. They often obsess about a perceived flaw in their appearance and become distressed and distracted by their body image. Needless to say, it's perfectly natural to want to look good, but what concerns me is how some people become vulnerable to this condition. Because we are multidimensional human beings, it's important to maintain a healthy balance and stay in tune with our body, mind, emotional, and spiritual states. If you feel that any of these four dimensions is being compromised, I highly recommend being resourceful and seeking professional advice. Actively taking good care of yourself, being mindful and soulful while being realistic and forgiving, means loving yourself and accepting the natural process of life. The key is to understand that "optimum" is relative and that at any given time there's so much to be grateful for. Start by counting your blessings and then address your challenges. Coming from love, acceptance, and gratitude is a timeless regimen for a healthier and more content life.

Actively taking good care of yourself, being mindful and soulful while being realistic and forgiving, means loving yourself and accepting the natural process of life.

The Importance of Your Microbiome

The very roots of your immune system lie in the microbiome. I've spent a lot of time reviewing the importance of the immune system to your overall health. Stem cells play an important role in our overall immune resilience. As you consider integrating stem cell therapy into your lifestyle, building and maintaining a healthy gut is an important factor in keeping your whole system working optimally. This means supporting a diverse and balanced gut microbiome, so that your gastrointestinal system can properly absorb essential nutrients and get rid of any toxins or waste that can interfere with metabolism. In this state of balance, you're much better at guarding your body from infection. However, an imbalance in the gut flora, the collection of bacteria that live in the gut for your benefit, can easily become overrun by microbes or too much bad bacteria. When there's a proliferation of bad bacteria and a dearth of good bacteria, the lining of the colon and intestines can become inflamed and vulnerable to infection. So how do you make sure your microbiome stays regulated and in healthy balance? You eat a low-acid or alkaline diet, make sure you eat enough fiber, drink plenty of water, and consume foods that act as pre- and probiotics to make sure that you have sufficient and varied flora (i.e., bacteria) to maintain balance.

Optimal Eating

Eating well does not have to be hard, and again, it comes down to balance. In general, my approach to eating starts with eating holistically, which means choosing as many whole foods as possible from all food groups and avoiding processed or packaged foods as much as possible. It may not come as a surprise that I enjoy eating and preparing Middle Eastern dishes. Both my wife and I come from food traditions that emphasize fresh vegetables like cucumbers, tomatoes, carrots, and peppers. We often enjoy salads that include vegetables and legumes, such as garbanzo beans, and dishes that include parsley, lemon, onions, and garlic for flavor. Another reason I enjoy and recommend Middle Eastern foods is that many dishes liberally incorporate spices and herbs, such as turmeric, saffron, and cumin, which not only enhance flavor but also are naturally anti-inflammatory.

The Mediterranean approach to eating is also well rounded and clean forward. Both of these traditions emphasize holistic eating by including fresh and natural foods, including olive oil, fruits, and vegetables, and avoiding processed foods.

But one point I try to drive home to all my patients and family members is to do their best to avoid industrialized foods that are processed or artificial; these foods are often full of sugars and have an acidic impact on the gut, causing inflammation and imbalance in our bodies. Instead, eat:

- lots of green, fibrous vegetables for sufficient fiber (green vegetables naturally contain a lot of fiber, as do legumes such as lentils and beans);
- more lemon, peppers, and spices that reduce acidity and inflammation in the body;
- moderate amounts of meat and fish (protein); and
- less refined sugars and fewer processed foods.

This approach to eating emphasizes whole foods and maintaining an optimal combination of protein, fats, carbohydrates, and fiber. Natural dietary fiber is key to helping maintain a healthy microbiome. Fiber moves food through the body and helps your gut stay in balance with the right amount and kinds of flora. Keep in mind that everyone's microbiome is different—there are no two alike, just as there are no two people completely alike. In addition to eating sufficient fiber, you can establish a healthy microbiome by drinking plenty of water to stay well hydrated, eating sufficient antioxidants to support the immune system's ability to get rid of toxins and waste, supporting a healthy gut with fermented foods and yogurt, and keeping your gut in pH balance—that is, with the right ratio of alkaline and acidic conditions.

The typical American diet—which is high in red meat, processed foods, and sugar—is associated with a highly acidic microbiome, leaky gut, and other inflammatory conditions affecting the lining of the GI tract. I suggest to patients that they think of their plate as an array of color: greens, yellows, and oranges. The more colorful, the more likely that their choices include lots of fruits and veggies! Whole fruit also contains important antioxidants (e.g., vitamin C), minerals (e.g., potassium), and fiber, so it's good to eat whole fruit in season and in moderation. Other factors to consider are the genetically modified products and pesticides on our products versus organic foods. Ayurveda adds the concepts of cooling and warming foods, and when and who should eat each.

Portion size depends on your body type, weight, and how much exercise you get on a regular basis. If you're hungry, then eat, but be mindful of how much. Again, moderation is a good rule to follow.

Finally, having routines is good for you as it allows the body to function in a healthy and controlled manner. Eating and sleeping times that are regular and predictable help balance your diurnal rhythms, hormones, and metabolism. (I'll go into the importance of sleep on overall body regulation in a moment.) Eating regularly helps your metabolism and metabolic cycle get into a rhythm. Some of my patients enjoy eating three meals like clockwork; other patients prefer to eat a big breakfast and a big dinner; still others choose to eat a late breakfast or brunch and dinner. I don't advise one way of timing your meals, but what I do recommend is establishing a routine—a routine that can be broken, of course, but one that anchors your metabolic clock. Your body's digestive system will begin to settle into a rhythm when meals are generally at the same time every day. This enables your metabolic system to be more efficient in terms of digestion, utilization of energy, and ultimately excretion.

In general, think of treating your body as an ecosystem. In order to make it function optimally, you want to give it clean, good foods that are satisfying and nutritionally beneficial. As I tell my patients, think of food as medicine, and the cleaner it is, the better.

Drink Plenty of Water

I'm sure you've heard the advice to drink plenty of water, so I doubt this is news to you. But it's still incredibly important to keep your body well hydrated. And while our needs for hydration vary with our bodies, the types of foods we eat (some foods, such as fruits and vegetables, contain water), and how much we exercise, drinking sufficient water is a must to help the microbiome stay in balance. Staying hydrated also helps your overall cellular health, blood circulation, digestion, and skin integrity and appearance. As we age, staying hydrated is vital in order to avoid suffering from many medical conditions that occur with dehydration, such as kidney damage and blood pressure problems.

As noted, some foods you eat contain water, including most fruits and vegetables. Processed foods, on the other hand, which are high in caffeine or sugars, deplete our bodies of fluid. I believe that dehydration, especially as we age, is a major contributor to strokes and organ damage.

So how much should you drink? The recommended eight 12-ounce glasses per day is wise. I'm a big fan of water with a squeeze of lemon; this combination provides both electrolytes and an acid-reducing effect on the gut at the same time.

Supporting Your Immune System with Functional Foods

Enhancing your health and positioning it to benefit optimally from stem cell therapy, whether that be through a procedure like the Stem Cell Lift or plant stem cell–derived products, in large part comes down to supporting your immune system. The immune system is made up of two distinct arms that work in tandem. On the one hand, the adaptive immune system acts like a defense system (characterized by B-cell and T-cell activity) and takes longer than the innate immune response to become active. The adaptive arm responds to pathogens or foreign agents that enter or threaten the body. In particular B cells produce specific antibodies to neutralize antigens (produced by the pathogen) or otherwise activate other aspects of the adaptive immune system to attack and destroy the foreign invaders.

The innate defense system works much more quickly and in a more generalized way, emitting different types of immune cells (such as macrophages, natural killer cells, and dendritic cells) to remove pathogens and then recruit other immune cells to fight against invaders. Overall, these innate immune cells are part of the first line of defense against external pathogens.

Why do I bring up these details about the immune system? Because you can strengthen both stem cells and these lifestyle elements to support your immune system, which in turn prevents disease and offsets aging. A 2022 article in *Nature* cited research that has shown—basically confirming what we have known all along—that the "consumption of specific functional foods can stimulate activity of immune cells, providing protection against cancer, viruses, and bacteria."[1]

In general, functional foods, containing bioactive compounds called nutraceuticals, are the fruits and vegetables that support your regenerative capacity to keep you healthy.

Certain foods have also been known to promote stem cell growth and health. These foods contain anti-inflammatory plant sterols and include cruciferous veggies such as cauliflower, broccoli, kale, cabbage, bok choy, garden cress, and Brussels sprouts.

Further, some supplements also have been shown to support the immune system and stem cell health, including:

- Carnosine
- Catechin
- Curcumin (found in turmeric)
- Fish oil
- NAD+
- Resveratrol
- Spirulina
- Vitamin C
- Vitamin D3

Here's a list of some natural whole foods that are functional:

- Vegetables: Broccoli, cauliflower, kale, spinach
- Fruits: Berries, kiwi, pears, peaches, apples, oranges, bananas
- Seeds: Chia seeds, flax seeds, hemp seeds, pumpkin seeds
- Nuts: Almonds, cashews, pistachios, macadamia nuts, Brazil nuts
- Legumes: Black beans, chickpeas, lentils
- Whole grains: Oats, barley, brown rice, couscous
- Seafood: Anchovies, cod, mackerel, salmon, sardines
- Fermented foods: Tempeh, kombucha, kimchi, kefir, sauerkraut
- Herbs and spices: Turmeric, cinnamon, ginger, cayenne pepper
- Beverages: Coffee, green tea, black tea

Research has established the clear immune-enhancing benefits of certain functional foods, including:

- Ginseng (white and red)
- Mushrooms, which are the fruit of fungi, such as *A. blazei*, reishi, maitake
- Chlorella, a type of green algae
- Probiotics, *L. plantarum*
- Green tea

These foods have been shown to support cancer therapy, contain antitumor benefits, and modulate the adaptive and innate immune systems.

As with any supplement, quality and quantity matters, so take the time to consider the reputation of the manufacturer, the sources of the active ingredients, and the concentrations provided in the suggested dosage. It's also important to check with your doctor for any contraindications if you are taking prescription medicines.

Exercise Stimulates Resilience

Sports and physical activity in childhood and young adulthood build strong bones and muscles that will serve you for the rest of your life. Most physical injuries occur when you lose muscle strength, flexibility, and balance. As you grow older, maintaining muscle strength and flexibility is vital to your health and to avoid injury.

Exercise is the intentional movement or physical activity that you do routinely. It may be cardiovascular, toning, or strengthening in nature. Exercise is essential for your physical, emotional, and mental health. It has been shown to improve mood, reduce stress and depression, and delay or minimize neurological deterioration such as dementia. Routine physical activity also keeps your cells healthy and in balance. It improves your immune function, your microvascular circulation, and the regenerative capacity of your stem cells. The more you move, the longer and better you live.

Exercise improves food absorption and therefore helps maintain weight; helps manage blood sugar and fights inflammation, both of which can prevent disease (such as type 2 diabetes); improves sleep; and literally energizes the body—the more you move, the more energy you feel! In my mind, there really is no downside to exercise.

That said, I also appreciate that for some people, getting into and sticking to a regular exercise routine is difficult. People have jobs, children, and lots of other responsibilities that get in the way of carving out time to exercise. So what's my solution? Walk!

If you're not already participating in a sport, going to the gym regularly, or working out in other ways, then walking is a wonderful option. Walking 30 minutes every day will have tremendous benefits for your mind, mood, and body by helping to regulate metabolism.

Of course, it's wise to check with your physician when beginning any new exercise routine, especially if you have a chronic condition. But in general, walking is safe, especially when you maintain a moderate pace and wear sensible shoes like sneakers. And walking doesn't require any kind of fancy equipment!

This simple and priceless activity can be most valuable and beneficial to your overall health and well-being.

Sleep Helps You Reset

We all know that babies and children need good sleep to develop optimally. But adults—especially as we age—also require good sleep. I know that when I am jet lagged or have not slept well, I cannot bring my A game to the day. Of course, I have high expectations of myself, but whenever this occurs, I'm reminded of how sensitive our brains and bodies are to sleep. As I help my patients prepare for the Stem Cell Lift procedure, I will sit down with them and discuss the importance of sleep to their healing. But sleep is just as important to optimal functioning and resisting illness.

Sleep enables your brain to clear out toxins that build up during the day; resets hormone and other neurochemical levels; consolidates your memories that are so important for learning and other cognitive functions; and protects you against illness and disease. Sleep is also paramount for regulating mood—as we can all attest after one or more bad nights of sleep that leave us feeling cranky and short-tempered.

Sleep for Regeneration

As you sleep, your body goes into regeneration mode. Your cells renew, repair, grow, and reset. This is why when you need the energy to grow or to heal from an illness, you sleep more. When you sleep well, your mind and body are in balance, and you feel rested, energized, sharp, and happy. Your body's internal biological clock has a diurnal (daily) rhythm, also known as circadian rhythm, to schedule and allocate resources to enable you to function optimally. Sunlight and darkness have a major influence on the physiologic and biologic functions that are set by your internal clock to be carried out, such as your sleep pattern, hormonal control and balance, and metabolism (including appetite and digestion).

Let's take a look at the sleep system to understand how best to optimize your sleep.

Understanding the Basics of Sleep

Sleep is either non-REM or REM, which refers to whether sleep includes dreams or not. In general, sleep is either light or deep and contains dreams or not. We cycle through four stages or states of sleep, with each stage presenting its own brain wave (as measured by an EEG) that reflects how much or little brain activity is happening.

Stage 1, for example, is relatively short and occurs when you first fall asleep; your heartbeat and breathing will slow, and your muscles relax.

Stage 2 is the longest sleep part of the sleep cycle; it's characterized by light sleep, a drop in body temperature, the cessation of eye movement, and slower brain wave activity.

Stage 3, also known as slow-wave sleep (SWS), marks a period of deep sleep and happens in the first half of the night; this is the type of sleep that's most acutely tied to the feeling we have of waking up refreshed. During stage 3 sleep, the body undergoes physical restoration and repair, such as muscle growth and tissue repair. This stage is also important for strengthening the immune system, which helps protect the body against infections and diseases.

During stage 4 sleep, or REM sleep, the brain processes and consolidates memories, which is important for learning and retaining information. It is also during this stage that the brain flushes out metabolic waste products that build up during waking hours, which may help prevent neurological disorders.

Overall, stages 3 and 4 are the most important for maintaining optimal health and well-being, and it is essential to get enough of both stages of sleep for overall health. Both stage 3 and stage 4 sleep are important for physical and mental health, and they serve different functions. In addition, the ideal proportion of stage 3 and stage 4 sleep varies from person to person and can change throughout the lifespan, but a healthy adult typically spends about 20 to 25 percent of their sleep time in SWS and about 20 to 25 percent of their sleep time in REM sleep. REM sleep is when your brain is most active (i.e., dreaming). Interestingly, during this period your heart rate and blood pressure resemble your typical daytime levels.

The Importance of Sleep Regulation

Sleep regulation does not have one particular physiological purpose, but rather is vital for our body's health overall, including

- Supporting proper growth and development
- Optimizing metabolism and utilization of energy
- Supporting the immune system
- Optimizing cognition
- Preventing disease
- Regulating mood

But living in a society where you are exposed to artificial light, technological noise, and distractions and travel through different time zones has exacerbated sleep dysregulation. As your body tries to maintain homeostasis, even during sleep, the cells of your body are taxed. Indeed, sleep disruption has been associated with such diseases as type 2 diabetes, cardiovascular disease, cancer, and intestinal disorders.

How to Improve Sleep

High-quality sleep is crucial to our overall health and well-being. The good news is that there's a lot of research going on in this field, and we are learning more and more about how sleep works and why it's so important. So let's return to our grounding concept of balance and consider a few simple ways to improve the quality of your sleep:

1. Try and go to bed at roughly the same time each night and wake around the same time each morning; establishing a regular sleep schedule will help regulate you in general.
2. Try to finish eating two to three hours before bedtime.
3. Keep caffeine to the early part of the day, avoiding it after 1 or 2 p.m. Caffeine is a stimulant and will affect your sleep-wake cycle.
4. Avoid screen time at least one hour before going to sleep and put your phone or other device far from your bed.

As you think about your current lifestyle, pay attention to what matters: that you eat holistically, exercise regularly, include some functional food supplements, and get good sleep. The key is to set attainable goals and implement sustainable routines. Awareness, moderation, and steady and gradual progress are usually more achievable and sustainable than radical and extreme changes, so be forgiving of yourself and celebrate small positive changes.

Pay attention to what matters: that you eat holistically, exercise regularly, include some functional food supplements, and get good sleep. The key is to set attainable goals and implement sustainable routines. Be forgiving of yourself and celebrate small positive changes.

Epilogue

A Paradigm Shift in Medicine Is on the Horizon

Because of their inherent plasticity, stem cells have become the focus of tremendous research. I am proud to be included in the group of dedicated scientists who understand and appreciate the potential of stem cell technology to advance medicine. As we all start to adopt regenerative science and technology to improve our health, well-being, and vitality, we as a society become educated about and embrace these advancements. As I continue to drive my research and clinical work, I believe strongly that this unique biotechnology has the potential to usher in a new paradigm for medicine, not only merging the fields of traditional and regenerative medicine but also offering hope to us all.

Transforming regenerative medicine for wellness and longevity, stem cell technology, to me, is a gift of the present and the promise of the near future!

Timeline of Dr. Nathan Newman's Stem Cell Journey of Discovery

1986	University of Southern California, 1986–1990 Research on novel UVA sunscreen at UCLA
1989	Scientific research published: • Substantivity of UVA sunscreens with Nicholas J. Lowe, MD, Clinical Professor of Dermatology, UCLA. • Current methods for testing chemicals for UVA efficacy (Parasol 1789) with Nicholas J. Lowe, MD, Clinical Professor of Dermatology, UCLA.
1990	Albert Einstein College of Medicine, Bronx, NY, 1990–1994 Founder and editor of the *Einstein Times*, a student publication, 1991–1993
1992	Scientific research published: • Newman N. Clinical improvement of photoaged skin with 50% glycolic acid: a double-blind, vehicle-controlled study. Presented to the American Society of Dermatologic Surgery, Scottsdale, Arizona.
1994	Medical degree (MD) Internship, Internal Medicine, UCLA-Wadsworth VA, West Los Angeles, CA, 1994–1995
1996	Residency, Dermatology, Cook County Hospital, Chicago, IL, 1996–1999 Scientific research published: • Newman N, Newman A, Moy LS, Babapour R, Harris AG. Clinical improvement of photoaged skin with 50% glycolic acid: A double-blind, vehicle-controlled study. *Dermatol Surg*. 1996;22:445–60.

1998	Scientific research published: • Landeck A, Newman N, Breadon L, Zahner S. A simple technique for ear piercing. *J Am Acad Dermatol.* 1998;39:795–6.
1999	Fellowship, Cosmetic Surgery, American Academy of Cosmetic Surgery, Riverside, CA, 1999–2000
2000	Established private practice, Beverly Hills, CA, 2000–present Regenerative Medicine, Stem Cells Research and Clinical Treatment, Cosmetic Surgery and Dermatology Founder and Medical Director, Orchid Outpatient Surgical and Medical Center, Inc., 2000–present
2001	Started to utilize autologous adipose (fat) stem cells in clinic. Scientific research published: • Shemer A, Nathansohn N, Kaplan B, Weiss G, Newman N, Trau H. Treatment of scalp seborrheic dermatitis and psoriasis with an ointment of 40% urea and 1% bifonazole. *Int J Dermatol.* 2000 Jul;39(7):532–4. • Eremia S, Newman N. Long-term follow-up after autologous fat grafting: Analysis of Results from 116 Patients Followed at Least 12 Months After Receiving the Last of a Minimum of Two Treatments. *Dermatol Surg.* 2000 Dec;26:1150–8. • Eremia S, Newman N. Topical anesthesia for laser hair removal: comparison of spot sizes and 755 nm versus 800 nm wavelengths. *Dermatol Surg.* 2000 Jul;26(7):667–9.
2009	Stem Cell Lift procedure trademarked Jeunesse Global launched with Luminesce skincare line
2010	Rinati Skin, LLC, established
2014	Authored three chapters in stem cell surgical textbook, *Stem Cells in Aesthetic Procedures: Art, Science, and Clinical Techniques* by Shiffman et al. (Springer, 2014): • Ear lobe revolumization (doi:10.1007/978-3-642-45207-9_33) • Stem cell enhanced fat grafting to buttocks (doi:10.1007/978-3-642-45207-9_43) • Hand rejuvenation (doi:10.1007/978-3-642-45207-9_47) Patents granted: • PAT. NO: 8,679,170: Methods and apparatus for therapeutic application of thermal energy • PAT. NO: 8821533: Device for minimally invasive plastic surgery lift procedure

2015	Scientific research published: • Newman N, Dolphin NN, Newman GR. Signs and symptoms of genital Lichen Sclerosus in women seeking autologous adipose derived stem cell treatment. *Med Obstet Gynecol.* 2015;3(4):1067. Patent granted: • PAT. NO: 9,066,781: Methods and apparatus for therapeutic application of thermal energy
2017	Scientific research published: • Newman N, Talavera-Adame D, Newman D. Conventional and novel stem cell-based therapies for androgenic alopecia. *Stem Cells Cloning.* 2017;101–9.
2018	Scientific research published: • Newman N, Rogowski N, Newman D, and Talavera-Adame D. Autologous adipose-derived stem cell treatment for women with genital Lichen Sclerosus. *J Gynecol Reprod Med.* 2018;2(4):1–4.
2019	Scientific research presented at the Annual Meeting of the International Society for Stem Cell Research (June 26–29, 2019) and published: • Talavera-Adame D, Rajangam A, Sidhu H, Khan N, Newman N. Consortia Factors Induce Differentiation of Adipose Stem Cells to Hair Follicle Stem Cells. Convention Center at Los Angeles, CA, USA. 2019 Annual Meeting of the International Society for Stem Cell Research. June 26–29, 2019. • Talavera-Adame D, Sidhu H, Rogowski N, Newman N. Comparative analysis of secretory factor profiles of human stromal vascular fraction by body region. Convention Center at Los Angeles, CA, USA. 2019 Annual Meeting of the International Society for Stem Cell Research. June 26–29, 2019. • Sidhu H, Talavera-Adame D, Newman N. Characterization of human adipose stem cells growing in optimized serum-free xeno-free media. Convention Center at Los Angeles, CA, USA. 2019 Annual Meeting of the International Society for Stem Cell Research. June 26–29, 2019.
2020	Scientific research published: • Talavera-Adame D, Sidhu H, Rogowski N, and Newman N. Comparative analysis of secretory factor profile of human stromal vascular fraction by body region. *American Journal of Translational Medicine* 2020; 4(2): 55–69.
2021	Scientific research published: • Sidhu H, Talavera-Adame D, Newman N. Characterization of primary and immortalized human adipose stem cells cultured in a novel serum-free xeno-free media. *American Journal of Translational Medicine* 2021; 5(2), 85–111.

2022	Patent granted: • PAT. NO: 11473117: System and method for the production, formulation and use of conditioned media, cultured cells and the factors included therein Aesthetic Management Partners (AMP Biologics) launched with EXO|E technology
2023	The STEM Company launched as a science-led platform pioneering plant-based cellular signaling solutions, with its first focus on topical regenerative skincare.
2025	Scientific research published: • Talavera-Adame, D., Palomares M, Plaza MR, Rogowski N, Lee BS, Zemach A, Newman, N. Novel. Reproducible, consortia factors derived from adipose stem cells for burn wound treatment. *Stem Cells Cloning* 2025; 18: 63–72. Patent granted: • Pat. NO: 16/839,031: System and method for production, formulation, and use of conditioned media, cultured cells and the factors included therein specific to the treatment of respiratory distress such as SARS-CoV, SARS-CoV2, or COVID-19.

Notes

Chapter 5

1 Nathan Newman, Nualla Rogowski, Daniella Newman, and Dodanim Talavera-Adame, "Autologous Adipose-Derived Stem Cell Treatment for Women with Genital Lichen Sclerosus," *Gynecology & Reproductive Health* 2, no. 4 (2018): 1–4, https://doi.org/10.33425/2639-9342.1052.

2 Sandra J. Gulin, Filippa Lundin, and Oliver Seifert, "Comorbidity in Patients with Lichen Sclerosus: A Retrospective Cohort Study," *European Journal of Medical Research* 28, no. 1 (2023): 338, https://doi.org/10.1186/s40001-023-01335-9.

3 Meng Zhao et al., "Age-Standardized Incidence, Prevalence, and Mortality Rates of Autoimmune Diseases in Adolescents and Young Adults (15–39 Years): An Analysis Based on the Global Burden of Disease Study 2021," *BMC Public Health* 24, no. 1 (2024): 1800, https://doi.org/10.1186/s12889-024-19290-3.

4 Mengjia Zhu et al., "Global, Regional, and National Burden of Inflammatory Bowel Disease in Older Adults: An Analysis of Data from the Global Burden of Disease Study 2021," *The Lancet*, https://ssrn.com/abstract=4924320.

5 Gabriel A. Gregory et al., "Global Incidence, Prevalence, and Mortality of Type 1 Diabetes in 2021 with Projection to 2040: A Modelling Study," *The Lancet: Diabetes & Endocrinology*, 10, no. 10 (2022): 741–760, https://doi.org/10.1016/S2213-8587(22)00218-2.

6 Global Asthma Network, "The Global Asthma Report 2022," http://globalasthmareport.org.

Chapter 6

1 World Health Organization, "Musculoskeletal Health," July 14, 2022, https://www.who.int/news-room/fact-sheets/detail/musculoskeletal-conditions.

Chapter 8

1 Dodanim Talavera-Adame, "Comparative Analysis of Secretory Factor Profiles of Human Stromal Vascular Fraction by Body Region," *American Journal of Translational Medicine* 4, no. 2 (2020), 55–69, https://journals3.publicknowledgeproject.org/index.php/ajtm/article/view/613

Chapter 9

1 Jae Hwan Kim, "Immunomodulatory Functional Foods and Their Molecular Mechanisms," *Experimental & Molecular Medicine* 54 (2022): 1–11, https://doi.org/10.1038/s12276-022-00724-0.

www.ingramcontent.com/pod-product-compliance
Lightning Source LLC
LaVergne TN
LVHW050912210926
848482LV00012B/408

* 9 7 9 8 2 1 8 7 9 9 4 7 2 *